Alzheimer's Early

What others are saying about this book…

"In *Alzheimer's Early Stages*, Dan Kuhn takes you gently but firmly by the hand and guides you into a better understanding of Alzheimer's disease. He offers you not only practical, clear, and compassionate strategies for coping with the myriad challenges you will face, but also philosophies for living life to the fullest with Alzheimer's. You will finish this book informed, reassured, inspired, and grateful. If you are reading anything about Alzheimer's disease, this book should be at the top of your pile."
— *Lisa Genova,* New York Times *bestselling author of* Still Alice

"I would highly recommend this book to our families that are dealing with a new diagnosis in an early-stage patient and also to professional caregivers working with patients in the early stages."
— *Daniel L. Paris, Massachusetts General Hospital, Memory Disorders Clinic*

"Dan Kuhn helps fill a void in the literature by offering families a wealth of insightful and practical information about early-stage Alzheimer's disease, something that too many families and patients have suffered through alone."
— *Mark A. Sager, MD, Professor of Medicine, University of Wisconsin Medical School and Director, Wisconsin Alzheimer's Institute*

"This essential book is for all family caregivers and friends of persons with early-stage Alzheimer's and the health-care providers who serve them. Not only are complex symptoms and treatment options discussed with much clarity, this book provides families helpful guidance in facing the challenges of adapting to and living with a new diagnosis. Dan Kuhn's book is an indispensable resource not only at the beginning, but throughout the course of the illness."
— *Darby Morhardt, PhD, Director of Education, Cognitive Neurology and Alzheimer's Disease Center, Northwestern University Feinberg School of Medicine*

"This well-written, thoughtful, and informative book should be on the shelf of every health-care provider and should also be recommended to those who are beginning their journey of caring for a person with Alzheimer's disease. Dan Kuhn is a knowledgeable, kind, and practical man, and readers will reap the benefits of his wisdom and sensitivity."
— *Mary S. Mittelman, DrPH, and Cynthia Epstein, MSW, New York University School of Medicine's Alzheimer's Disease Center and coauthors of* Counseling the Alzheimer's Caregiver: A Resource for Healthcare Professionals

"This uniquely thoughtful, practical, and encouraging book is an essential resource for any care partner beginning on an Alzheimer's path. Dan Kuhn's wise yet realistic messages provide the reassuring guidance and comfort needed to diffuse the fear and uncertainly that so often surround this challenging diagnosis."

— *Lisa Snyder, LCSW, Director of Quality of Life Programs,*
UC San Diego Shiley–Marcos Alzheimer's Disease Research Center;
author of Living Your Best with Early-Stage Alzheimer's *and*
Speaking Our Minds: What It's Like to Have Alzheimer's

"*Alzheimer's Early Stages* presents thoughtful, practical guidance for caregivers based on up-to-date scientific studies. The information provided is of the highest quality, and the guidance offered is thoroughly wise."

— *Stephen G. Post, PhD, author of* The Moral Challenge of Alzheimer Disease

"*Alzheimer's Early Stages* is a must-have book for anyone diagnosed with the disease and his or her family members. Thoughtful, informative, and wide ranging, it answers the questions many of us have when facing this challenging disease."

— *David Troxel, MPH, and Virginia Bell, MSW, co-authors of*
A Dignified Life: The Best Friends Approach to Alzheimer's Care

"Dan Kuhn's clear-eyed and full-hearted words are the ideal companion for those many millions who will experience memory loss in the coming decade. Read it yourself, and then have a stack of them ready to give to friends."

— *Anne Basting, PhD, author of* Forget Memory:
Creating Better Lives for People with Dementia

"*Alzheimer's Early Stages* provides a wealth of helpful information in a beautifully balanced manner and is relentlessly person-centered and positive. With great sensitivity, insight, and wisdom gained from years of experience, Dan Kuhn has updated this important resource for all whose lives are confronted by the reality of the changing mind."

— *G. Allen Power, MD, author of* Dementia Beyond Drugs:
Changing the Culture of Care

"Dan Kuhn offers thoughtful readers whose lives are touched by Alzheimer's disease an excellent resource for information about the disease process itself, with a particularly fine section on the lived experience, ways to plan for and enhance daily life as well as essential information about caring for the self."

— *Carol Bowlby Sifton, BA BscOT, author of*
Navigating the Alzheimer's Journey

Selected Reviews of Earlier Editions

"…an Alzheimer's classic to be sure. A must-have for the well-read persons interested in Alzheimer's disease."

— *American Journal of Alzheimer's Disease*

"Kuhn guides families in developing a philosophy of care, offering clear and current information on the nature of the illness…this is a much needed addition to the Alzheimer's literature."

— *Library Journal*

"*Alzheimer's Early Stages* is practical, authoritative, and written with a clarity that will be appreciated by the general reader."

— *Reviewer's Bookwatch*

"Daniel Kuhn…writes with calm authority about a disease that is legendary for creating fear, confusion, and loneliness. His approach is realistic but reassuring."

— *The Birmingham News*

"…[the author's] hands-on experience with and empathy for persons with dementia and their caregivers jump off the page in this impressive new book."

— *Early Alzheimer's: A Forum for Early Stage Dementia Care*

"…does a sensitive and comprehensive job of addressing the medical, emotional, and practical concerns inherent in the early stages…. It is a valuable addition to the Alzheimer's literature and Mr. Kuhn is to be commended for this very worthwhile contribution."

— *Perspectives: A Newsletter for Individuals with Alzheimer's or a Related Disorder*

"Daniel Kuhn's book is a welcome addition to the caregiver literature."

— *Family Caregiver Alliance* newsletter

"…highly recommended as a state-of-the-art review on managing the disease and the people who care for them. No social worker's library should be without Kuhn's book."

— *Journal of Social Work in Long-Term Care*

"Dan Kuhn has been listening to persons with [Alzheimer's disease] and their families throughout his many years of practice and has put this understanding to good use in this book. Social workers will be pleased to have this excellent resource to recommend to their clients."

— *Social Work AGEnda, Newsletter of the Association for Gerontology in Social Work*

Ordering

Trade bookstores in the U.S. and Canada please contact
Publishers Group West
1700 Fourth Street, Berkeley CA 94710
Phone: (800) 788-3123   Fax: (800) 351-5073

For bulk orders please contact
Special Sales
Hunter House Inc., PO Box 2914, Alameda CA 94501-0914
Phone: (510) 899-5041   Fax: (510) 865-4295
E-mail: sales@hunterhouse.com

Individuals can order our books by calling **(800) 266-5592**
or from our website at **www.hunterhouse.com**

Alzheimer's Early Stages

First Steps for Families, Friends and Caregivers

THIRD EDITION

DANIEL KUHN, MSW

Hunter House
PUBLISHERS

Grateful acknowledgment is made for permission to reprint excerpts from the following works: *My Journey into Alzheimer's Disease* by Robert Davis, Wheaton, IL: Tyndale House Publishers, 1989; *Living in the Labyrinth* by Diana Friel McGowin, Forest Knolls, CA: Elder Books, 1994; *Show Me the Way to Go Home* by Larry Rose, Forest Knolls, CA: Elder Books, 1995; *Who Will I Be When I Die?* by Christine Boden, East Melbourne, Australia: HarperCollins Publishers, 1998; *Partial View: An Alzheimer's Journal* by Cary Smith Henderson, Ruth D. Henderson, and Jackie H. Main, Dallas, TX: Southern Methodist University Press, 1998. *All rights reserved.*

Library of Congress Cataloging-in-Publication Data
Kuhn, Daniel.
Alzheimer's early stages : first steps for family, friends and caregivers /
Daniel Kuhn. — Third edition.
pages   cm
Includes bibliographical references and index.
ISBN 978-0-89793-667-5 (trade paper) — ISBN 978-0-89793-668-2 (ebook)
1. Alzheimer's disease — Popular works.   2. Caregivers.   I. Title.
RC523.2.K838 2013
616.8'31 — dc23   2013010345

Project Credits

Cover Design: Jinni Fontana	Special Sales Manager: Judy Hardin
Book Production: John McKercher	Rights Coordinator: Candace Groskreutz
Copy Editor: Amy Bauman	Publisher's Assistant: Bronwyn Emery
Indexer: Nancy D. Peterson	Customer Service Manager: Christina Sverdrup
Managing Editor: Alexandra Mummery	Order Fulfillment: Washul Lakdhon
Editorial Intern: Jordan Collins	Administrator: Theresa Nelson
Acquisitions Intern: Sally Castillo	Computer Support: Peter Eichelberger
Publicity Coordinator: Martha Scarpati	Publisher: Kiran S. Rana

Printed and bound by Sheridan Books, Ann Arbor, Michigan
Manufactured in the United States of America

9 8 7 6 5 4 3 2 1   Third Edition   13 14 15 16 17

Contents

Part I: What Is Alzheimer's Disease?

Part II: Giving Care

Foreword

For over twenty-five hundred years, people have recognized that old age can be accompanied by the loss of memory and other cognitive abilities. However, Alzheimer's disease and other chronic conditions of aging have not been considered a public health problem until recently. This is mainly the result of the remarkable increase in life expectancy that has been achieved during the past century. With people living longer and fertility declining, both the number and percentage of the older population continues to increase rapidly. This "silver tsunami" will continue well into the twenty-first century. The recognition of these demographic changes led to the founding of the National Institute on Aging in 1976 and the funding of the first Alzheimer's disease research centers in the United States in 1985.

But even with this increased attention to the problem, only a fraction of the estimated five million Americans with Alzheimer's disease currently come to the attention of the health-care system. The majority are living at home, alone or with families, slowly developing memory problems but not seeking help. In these cases a sort of conspiracy exists between the person with the disease, their family and friends, and their physician. There is a silent agreement not to talk about the memory problems until the disease has progressed to a more advanced stage, when the signs and symptoms cannot be concealed and the condition cannot be denied. Unfortunately, this conspiracy results in the loss of precious time that could have been used to avoid crises, plan for the future, involve the person with the disease in decision making, and treat the signs and symptoms of the illness.

Why is there so much resistance to recognizing, acknowledging, and confronting Alzheimer's disease in an open and forthright manner? The answer is complicated, but this reticence is partly due to fear. For years, Alzheimer's disease has been dramatized as a disease that steals the mind, destroys the ability to recognize family and friends, leads to an inability to control bodily functions, changes personality, and ultimately results in institutionalization and death. However, the disease does not develop overnight. You do not wake up in the morning with Alzheimer's disease, as would be the case with a stroke or heart attack. Alzheimer's is an insidious disease. In the words of Daniel Kuhn, "the disease is like an unwelcome stranger that creeps into the lives of everyone it visits." Furthermore, the disease is not necessarily a death sentence or a harbinger of a stark reality worse than death. A simple fact is that the majority of people with Alzheimer's disease are old, have a mild form, and die from something else before the disease progresses to more severe stages.

Now that the dramatic images of Alzheimer's disease have captured the attention of scientists, laypeople, and politicians, it is time to think about how the disease begins. Alzheimer's disease has a beginning, not just an end. Much has been learned about the disease since the U.S. government invested in the first Alzheimer's disease research centers, and much has been learned since the second edition of this book appeared a decade ago. The disease is now recognized as a chronic, age-related disease. Like other chronic diseases of aging, it has a long pre-clinical period during which the pathology develops without signs or symptoms. This is followed by a mild cognitive impairment during which cognitive abilities are compromised but affected people remain highly functional. Finally, there is the appearance of Alzheimer's-type dementia.

Since the last edition of this book a number of biological markers of the disease have been developed. Spinal fluid tests have been developed that can identify amyloid and tau, the two key constituents of brain pathology. Amyloid can also be imaged with positron emission tomography (PET) scans. These tests are being incorporated into clinical trials of persons with very early Alzheimer's disease, long before the onset of dementia. However, they are not yet used in clinical practice.

Since the last edition of this book, the results of the human genome project have yielded dividends for Alzheimer's disease. We have now identified about a dozen genetic risk factors for the disease. They are providing new clues into the biological beginnings of Alzheimer's disease and new leads on potential novel therapies. However, these too are not yet used in clinical practice.

Since the last edition of this book, epidemiologic studies have provided us with a wide range of lifestyle factors that appear to influence risk of disease. Thus, a lifestyle that includes active engagement in cognitive, physical, social, leisure, and emotionally rewarding activities may forestall or slow age-related cognitive decline.

Unfortunately, however, since the last edition of this book there has not been a single new drug approved by the U.S. Food and Drug Administration for the treatment or prevention of Alzheimer's disease. Thus, much more needs to be learned about the disease.

Treating and preventing Alzheimer's disease will take four things. First, it takes dedicated groups of researchers. Second, it takes dedicated volunteers including patients and families, and healthy older adults, to participate in a wide range of studies. Third, it takes money—lots of money. Preventing Alzheimer's disease will be expensive. The current U.S. National Institutes of Health budget for research on the disease is about $500 million annually, a small fraction of what is spent on research for cancer and heart disease. The latter conditions are devastating and deserve every penny of funding, but Alzheimer's disease is also devastating. Finally, it takes time—human studies of the disease take years to complete.

This book strives to educate the reader about what we know and what we have learned about Alzheimer's disease. It will bring you up to date with medical research. It will also share with you the latest thoughts about the care of people with the disease from a highly experienced social worker who has been at the forefront of the disease for decades. Dan Kuhn has been working with older people with Alzheimer's disease and other age-related conditions for more than forty years. For over a dozen years he performed this valuable work at the Rush Alzheimer's Disease Center in Chicago, a large multidisciplinary center devoted to research, education, and care that is supported by the Illinois Department of Public Health and the National Institute on Aging. Following work at Mather LifeWays Institute on Aging and the Alzheimer's Association, he now continues his efforts at Rainbow Hospice and Palliative Care.

This book reflects Dan's considerable experience, wisdom, and thoughtfulness. He has directly improved the lives of many people with Alzheimer's disease and their loved ones. It is with great pride that I see his knowledge shared with those who have not had the good fortune to work with him directly. I sincerely hope that through this book, Dan will be able to reach out and improve the lives of many more people with Alzheimer's disease, as well as the lives of their families and friends.

— David A. Bennett, MD, Director,
Rush Alzheimer's Disease Center
Rush University Medical Center, Chicago

Acknowledgments

I am indebted to many people for their inspiration and help in writing the three editions of this book. Heartfelt thanks to my former colleagues at the Rush Alzheimer's Disease Center, especially Anna Ortigara, Carly Hellen, Dorothy Seman, Dr. Jacob Fox, Dr. Concetta Forchetti, and Dr. David Bennett. I am also grateful to my former colleagues at Mather LifeWays Institute on Aging, especially Bill Keane, Joni Gatz-Bauman, Dr. David Lindeman, Dr. Linda Hollinger-Smith, Dr. Brad Fulton, Dr. Perry Edelman, and the late Kathleen Ustick. I also owe much thanks to my former colleagues at the Alzheimer's Association, especially Susan Rothas, Nicole Batsch, and Courtney Bayron. Thanks, too, to my current colleagues at Rainbow Hospice and Palliative Care, especially Amy Frazier, Pat Ahern, and Dr. Jeannine Forrest.

I am also grateful for the many professionals and friends who share my personal mission to improve the care of people with Alzheimer's disease and their families, especially Lisa Snyder, David Troxel, Virginia Bell, Mike Denesha, Julie Lamberti, Tena Alonzo, Juliet Holt, Dr. Darby Morhardt, Dr. Maribeth Gallagher, Dr. Carol Long, Dr. Dawn Brooker, the late Dr. Tom Kitwood, and the staff of The Retirement Research Foundation.

Thanks to my beloved parents, Bill and Elaine Kuhn, who continue to be my greatest cheerleaders. Also, to my children, Curtis, Elizabeth, and Peter, who always give me reason to smile and be proud. May their children someday read about Alzheimer's disease in history books. In the meantime, may all of us create a better world for every person whose memories are fading away.

Finally, I am thankful to those countless men and women living with Alzheimer's disease who have graciously shared their joys and sorrows with me. You have taught me that the human spirit is untouched by this disease. I am humbled and amazed by your courage.

Introduction:
Why a Third Edition
of this Book?

This book is intended to serve as a beginning guide for family members and friends of people in the early stages of Alzheimer's disease. Although many fine books about Alzheimer's disease have been published, this was the first one written exclusively about its early stages, and it will hopefully continue to be a valued resource for everyone who confronts this disease. The latest medical information about the disease is explained, including new definitions about the disease itself, new diagnostic techniques, as well as current and proposed treatments. Practical advice about coping with the disease now and help in planning for the future are also offered. My goal is to shed light on the concerns of family members and friends who are newcomers to this troubling disease. If you have a relative or friend who has recently been diagnosed with Alzheimer's disease, this book aims to help you deal with the challenges at hand. Also, if you know someone who is having difficulties with memory, thinking, language, and other brain functions, I hope this book will encourage you to seek help for that individual.

For a variety of reasons, Alzheimer's disease is one of the most feared diseases today. It is often characterized only in the grimmest terms, and anyone who is just beginning to learn about Alzheimer's disease can get caught up in this doom and gloom. The disease is like an unwelcome stranger that creeps into the lives of everyone it visits.

It helps to get to know this stranger sooner rather than later, because it will not go away. Although life often becomes stressful for those who provide care and supervision, it is possible to successfully make adjustments. There is much life to be lived with Alzheimer's disease.

The beginning of Alzheimer's is a critical time to develop a philosophy of care and ways of coping that will promote a good quality of life both for the person with the disease and for his or her family and friends. Once you are armed with the information and advice offered in this book, hope and self-confidence can replace worry and fear. Becoming familiar with the disease in its initial stages will also help you prevent or minimize crises later on. Although knowledge is power in dealing with Alzheimer's disease, it is not enough to cope successfully. Learning to accept a lifestyle characterized by a "new normal" is also required. You can slowly adapt until new routines become habit and new challenges are not surprising, despite the progressive nature of the disease. Although flexibility and optimism will not alter the course of the disease, these skills can influence a healthy adaptation and empower you and other people to provide the best possible care for those with the disease.

For four decades I have been privileged to hear the stories of thousands of individuals with the disease, as well as stories from their relatives and friends. In unique ways, these people have expressed their thoughts and feelings about coming to terms with this life-changing experience. These men and women have been my best teachers, and I am grateful to them for how much they have taught me about living with this disease. An important lesson I have learned is that there is no single right way of coping. Therefore, this book is not a step-by-step guide to the "correct" or "best" way to manage the inherent challenges of this disease. Rather, throughout this book I address general principles about coping strategies and then offer specific suggestions. Whenever possible, I rely on the experiences of others familiar with Alzheimer's disease to illustrate key points.

When I began my career as a medical social worker in the 1970s, older people who were profoundly forgetful were labeled as "senile" or diagnosed by physicians as having "senile dementia" or "organic brain syndrome." Middle-age people who exhibited similar problems were diagnosed with a rare brain disorder known as "Alzheimer's disease." In the 1980s a seismic shift occurred when forgetfulness commonly associated with old age and the rare medical problem seen in middle age were firmly established as one and the same—Alzheimer's disease. The Alzheimer's Association and the National Institute on Aging began to raise public awareness and fund research into its causes, treatment, cure, and prevention. With the growing number of older persons in the 1990s, Alzheimer's disease became a known phrase. But the disease was still shrouded in mystery at the personal, societal, and medical levels.

The first edition of this book was published in 1999, shortly after the first drug treatments for Alzheimer's disease were developed. Although these new drugs were imperfect, there was much hope for further medical improvements. The second edition of this book was published in 2003, when promising research was believed to be paving the way toward medical breakthroughs. That hope has since given way to the reality that Alzheimer's disease is far more complex and stubborn than most scientists had imagined. No new drugs have been approved for treating the disease in the past ten years, amidst more than a hundred failures of experimental drugs tested in large clinical trials.

Today more than five million Americans have the disease, and it is projected that nearly fourteen million will have the disease by 2050 in the absence of prevention. Without question, progress is being made to understand the underlying biological mechanisms of Alzheimer's disease. There have also been advancements in identifying the disease in its earliest stages through improved diagnostic techniques. The first study focused on preventing the disease is now being launched in the most unlikely place—in Columbia, South America, where a rare gene has plagued a large, extended family whose members develop symptoms of the disease in middle age but whose brains begin to show microscopic damage decades earlier. It will take many years before the results of this first prevention study involving three novel drugs will be known and if any benefits can be applied to other people. Glimmers of hope can be also seen in the National Alzheimer's Project Act signed into law by President Barack Obama in 2011, which is a blueprint for research and services to help those affected by the disease. However, funding this ambitious plan will take political will and popular support to compete with other national priorities.

In the meantime, what can be done to live life to the fullest with Alzheimer's disease? In this book, I describe current and proposed medical treatments as well as many strategies for improving quality of life that can be easily used by family members and friends. I also speculate how new research about reducing potential risks for developing the disease can be used to slow progression and maximize quality of life for all concerned. I want to be clear: there are no proven ways to prevent the disease or slow down the progression of the disease, apart from a handful of imperfect drugs. We have tantalizing clues based upon research that deserve closer scrutiny. For example, the first U.S. government–sponsored study to test the potential benefits of physical exercise will begin soon. We also have loads of anecdotal reports about potential means of prevention and treatment that may prove useful or may turn out to be nothing more than quackery. These, too, are addressed in this updated edition.

Although every stage of the disease is difficult, the early phases can actually be the most troublesome because of ignorance and misinformation. My goal in this book is to provide hope to those who feel puzzled, worried, frightened, or overwhelmed by the presence of this stranger in their lives. Perhaps some insights drawn from the collective wisdom of others can help you meet the challenges you face now and prepare you for the future. Although the chance of a miracle cure being discovered any time soon is minute, you can find the grace to persevere in the midst of adversity.

How This Book Is Organized

Part I of this book concerns the medical aspects of Alzheimer's disease. This knowledge about basic medical facts will help you begin dealing with practical, everyday issues. Although three chapters are full of facts about diagnosis and treatment, you should not be too concerned about absorbing all of the details right away. A medical understanding of Alzheimer's is useful, but the living challenges posed by the disease are far more difficult to master. The final chapter in this section addresses the limits of medicine and emphasizes nonmedical ways to enhance the quality of life of someone with the disease. Part II addresses these day-to-day concerns including the emotional, social, legal, and financial effects of the disease on you, on your family and friends, and, above all, on your loved one with the disease. Understanding your changing roles and responsibilities in relation to the person with the disease is central to this undertaking. Part III specifically addresses how to best take care of yourself as you care for your loved one. Achieving a balance between your needs and the needs of the person with the disease is key to coping successfully. The epilogue lays out an agenda for change in public policy concerning research into the treatment and prevention of Alzheimer's disease. It also offers suggestions in the event that you wish to add your voices to the growing number of activists advocating for increased funding for research and improved services for everyone directly affected by Alzheimer's. Finally, there is a resource section that will direct you to helpful books, videos, websites, and organizations.

A note about the book's title: Although primarily addressed to caring for people with Alzheimer's disease, this book may well apply to individuals and families coping with a variety of other irreversible brain disorders. The term *early stages* refers to the fact that the disease unfolds over many years, perhaps decades as new research shows. My use of the word *stages* is an attempt to indicate that you will face different challenges along the continuum of the disease. Also, I have avoided using terms like *patient, victim,* or *sufferer,* and instead refer to the *person* or *people* with Alzheimer's disease. Maintaining one's humanity in the face of this dehumanizing disease is perhaps the greatest challenge for everyone involved, and we need to use language that upholds personhood and dignity. I have also avoided the term *caregiver* in describing family and friends who care for a person with the disease. You were first in a relationship with someone who now is experiencing a disabling condition. Your role in giving care is secondary to your personal relationship. The term *care partner* better describes both your past and present role in relation to the person with Alzheimer's disease. Your commitment, knowledge, skill, creativity, flexibility, resourcefulness, and faith are essential in meeting the many challenges that this disease presents to you now and in the future. I pray that this book can help you in taking the first important steps on this life-changing journey.

PART I

What Is Alzheimer's Disease?

1 The Need for an Accurate Diagnosis

It is evident that we are dealing with a peculiar, little-known disease process.

Alois Alzheimer, 1906

Aging is a process of change. As we grow older, our bodies gradually change in a variety of ways. Our hair may turn gray or start to thin. Our ears may lose their sensitivity to certain sounds. Our eyes may no longer see as well as they used to. Our skin wrinkles, and our muscle tone diminishes. Physical functions, in general, start to slow down. Older men are at greater risk of developing prostate problems than they were earlier in life. Older women are at greater risk of developing osteoporosis. Mental functions often slow down, too. Memory loss is fairly common and "senior moments" are taken for granted. We have grown accustomed to the fact that older people eventually become ill or frail. In other words, these changes occur naturally with advancing age. But should all such changes be considered normal just because they are common? Should we simply resign ourselves to living with the illnesses and disabilities associated with growing older? Most people facing the prospect of decline in old age would answer such questions with a resounding "No!"

A century ago, an American's average life span was fifty-two years, but now it has reached seventy-eight. What accounts for this dramatic change in longevity that has resulted in an aging boom today? As a society, we began to believe that life-threatening diseases could be treated, cured, and prevented. Improvements in public health during the past century altered our expectations. Lifestyle changes and medical breakthroughs have made a long life a reality for the average person in developed countries. In other words, there is no need today to think that disabling conditions associated with aging are "normal" just because they are commonplace. Such a shift in our thinking and our medical technology has spawned a large and growing "anti-aging" movement in health, fitness, and medicine.

What Is Normal and Abnormal in the Brain?

Forgetfulness is a universal human experience. For most of us, forgetting something represents nothing more than a temporary inconvenience, since usually the forgotten bits of information are trivial. Although advancing age typically brings about minor changes in memory, thinking, and other brain functions, most older adults tend to compensate quite well for these changes. And although older people may generally be more forgetful than they were in their younger years, this level of forgetfulness usually does not interfere with the overall quality of their lives. This condition is referred to as "benign forgetfulness." Although the majority of older people experience this minor problem, the scientific basis for this change late in life is not yet completely understood. Although most people aged sixty-five years and older experience a slight decline in memory and other brain functions, less than 15 percent decline in significant ways. Older people may occasionally complain about forgetting names or misplacing things around the home. They may also notice these incidents occur with greater regularity as they age. These moments of absent-mindedness do not seriously affect one's lifestyle and may simply be an exaggeration of forgetfulness experienced by everyone, regardless of age. Most of these people would perform very well on tests of memory and thinking if medically evaluated.

At first glance, age-related forgetfulness may appear similar to the forgetfulness associated with Alzheimer's disease (hereafter referred to as "AD"). If this is the case, then what exactly is the difference between these two states, one considered a normal part of aging and the other a sign of disease? There is currently no single test available that provides a clear answer to this basic question. A diagnosis of AD cannot yet be made with a simple biological test; it requires that certain "clinical" criteria be met, based on one's symptoms, such as memory loss worse than expected for one's age. Advances in brain science are offering important insights into the differences between AD and the earliest stages of the disease.

It is now commonly understood that memory loss and other cognitive impairments can be traced on a continuum between "normal" and "disease"—differences are merely a matter of degree. For someone who is actually experiencing memory problems, however, there is a notable difference between mild memory loss that is merely annoying and severe memory loss that disrupts one's life. For example, it is trivial to forget what foods one ate at a restaurant last night, but it is a serious problem to forget that one ate at a restaurant at all. When memory problems become severe enough that someone cannot live independently, then this degree of forgetfulness is indeed not normal. The subtle differences between mild memory loss and severe memory loss are part of that continuum. Unfortunately, the points along the continuum from "normal" to "disease" cannot yet be accurately defined 100 percent of the time. The good news is that standardized tests currently under development are likely to be in widespread clinical use by physicians in the near future.

A person who is experiencing persistent forgetfulness but no other apparent difficulty with thinking abilities may have a condition called "mild cognitive impairment."[1] This term, commonly referred to as "MCI," describes a stage between the benign forgetfulness commonly experienced by older people and the more trying and chronic problems associated with AD or a related brain disorder. MCI is characterized by mild decline in memory and other brain functions such as concentration and orientation. Someone with MCI may appear "normal" and be capable of carrying out complex tasks and living independently. Most concerning is that MCI often represents the very earliest stages of AD. Solid evidence now exists that the underlying biological processes that cause MCI are, in fact, the same processes that cause AD. Many individuals with MCI remain stable and remain independent with little or no assistance from others. However, a majority of these people worsen in their abilities over time, eventually crossing the threshold to the early stages of AD.

Psychological tests are available to help distinguish such mild impairments both from "normal aging" and from AD. However, such tests are not always precise. New biological tests that can identify abnormalities in one's blood or spinal fluid may soon become available to better differentiate MCI from other points along the continuum. Brain imaging tests now in development using magnetic resonance imaging (MRI) and positron emission tomography (PET) scans show great promise for differentiating points along the continuum. In the meantime, four indicators are being used by physicians to make a diagnosis of MCI:[2]

1. concern about a change in one's cognition functions, such as memory and problem solving, relative to previous functioning

2. impairment of one or more cognitive functions that is greater than expected for the person's age and education

3. preserved ability to function independently in daily life, though some complex tasks may be more difficult than before

4. no dementia (no interference with the ability to work or do usual activities)

Many physicians are treating people with MCI using the same drugs currently prescribed for AD, although no treatments have been approved for MCI. The fact that MCI is labeled a "medical condition" that is likely to lead to a full-blown "disease" may minimize how disruptive MCI is for all concerned. Families and friends of people with MCI face challenges similar to those faced every day by people coping with AD, except on a milder scale. The symptoms of MCI need to be taken seriously, regardless of how mild or benign they may seem at first glance. MCI is troubling, but it does not mean that one's quality of life should diminish. Adapting to this condition is necessary to continue enjoying life to the fullest. People with MCI may wish to enroll in research studies to find ways of slowing down the typical progression into AD.

Thus far, no definitive tests are available to determine when a person with MCI crosses the threshold to AD. Therefore, scientists have established criteria to make the distinction.[3] The criteria for AD include the following:

1. cognitive or behavioral symptoms of dementia that interfere with one's ability to work or do usual activities

2. symptoms that represent a decline from one's previous level of functioning

3. symptoms that have a gradual onset spanning months to years; they do not come on suddenly in a span of hours or days

4. a clear-cut history of worsening of cognition that is reported or observed

5. symptoms that are not explained by delirium (acute, short-term confusion due to another medical condition) or a major psychiatric disorder

6. cognitive or behavioral impairment that is detected through a combination of history-taking from the person with symptoms and a knowledgeable informant such as a family member and an objective cognitive assessment, through either a brief mental status examination or a battery of psychological testing

7. cognitive or behavioral impairment is present, involving a minimum of two of the following problems:

   a. impaired ability to acquire and remember new information

   b. impaired reasoning and handling of complex tasks

   c. impaired ability to recognize faces or common objects

   d. impaired language

   e. changes in personality, behavior, or comportment

With the help of these criteria, physicians who are experienced in assessing people with memory disorders such as AD are able to make an accurate clinical diagnosis in the majority of cases, but only after death can this diagnosis be fully confirmed through examination of brain tissue. People who meet the above criteria for a diagnosis of AD sometimes have other types of brain diseases or injuries instead of AD that need to be considered. For example, someone who has experienced small or silent strokes may show cognitive or behavioral changes similar to the symptoms of AD. A specialist is usually helpful when differentiating between types of irreversible brain disorders.

In 2011 the National Institutes of Health and the Alzheimer's Association announced new guidelines for distinguishing AD, MCI, and a "pre-clinical" stage.[4] These three distinct stages compose what is believed to represent the entire continuum of the disease. Figure 1.1 illustrates these stages, with cognitive functions like memory gradually declining over time. Prior to the onset of symptoms associated with either MCI or AD, subtle changes occur at a microscopic level deep within the brain. These changes are likely to lead to "full-blown" disease many years, or perhaps even decades, later. In this "pre-clinical" disease stage, key biological changes are under way in the body, but the disease has not yet caused any noticeable "clinical" symptoms. The concept of a pre-clinical stage of disease is well established. For example, high cholesterol can result in narrowing of the arteries that is detectible prior to a heart attack. Diabetes and high blood pressure are frequently detected through laboratory tests, and effective treatment can prevent the emergence of symptoms.

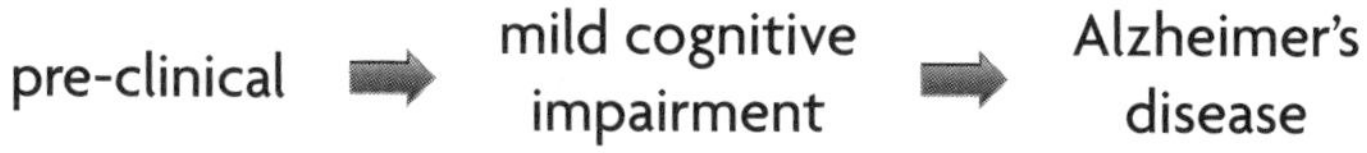

pre-clinical ➡ mild cognitive impairment ➡ Alzheimer's disease

FIGURE 1.1 The three stages of the disease continuum

The new guidelines do not include specific criteria for diagnosis of this pre-clinical stage. However, it is clear that progress is being made to identify "biomarkers" that may signal when these changes in the brain begin. Biomarkers, such as those sought for AD, are benchmarks in the body that can be reliably measured to indicate the presence or absence of a disease, or the likelihood of later developing a disease. For example, one's blood glucose level is a biomarker for diabetes, and one's blood cholesterol level is a biomarker for heart disease. Something tangible like these simple tests would be useful to definitively make a diagnosis of AD.

The strongest biomarker candidates for AD include brain imaging studies using MRI and PET scans. Tiny brain abnormalities known as amyloid plaques and neurofibrillary tangles, which were first identified by Dr. Alzheimer more than a century ago, can now be visualized many years before the onset of symptoms with the aid of these brain imaging techniques. In particular, a new chemical agent can identify amyloid plaques using a PET scan but this test is not yet capable of offering 100 percent certainty to a diagnosis of AD. In addition, abnormal protein levels in cerebrovascular fluid (CSF) show promise for detecting AD at all points on the continuum: pre-clinical, MCI, and AD. Simple blood tests are also under development for early detection of AD. Since none of these tests is completely reliable yet, they are not available for widespread, commercial use. And these tests are not yet being paid for by insurance. However, they are being used in research studies to identify people at risk of developing MCI and AD in order to test medical and behavioral interventions aimed at slowing progression.

In addition to the plaques and tangles that are the hallmark features of AD inside the brain, there is mounting evidence that other illnesses may harm the brain. It is estimated that more than half of people with AD also have damaged blood vessels in the brain, due to tiny strokes or cerebrovascular disease. How such damage interacts with the presence of AD plaques and tangles is unclear but the combination is deadly for brain cells. Brain imaging techniques noted above are often useful in identifying the presence of tiny strokes that may be contributing to symptoms associated with AD. Other disorders affecting the brain may also contribute to the onset or worsening of AD symptoms. Some of these brain disorders may be easily detected whereas others may be undetectable with present medical technology.

What about Genetic Testing?

We inherit a set of genes from both our mother and father that may protect us or put us at risk for certain diseases. Some defective genes or mutations can directly cause diseases such as cystic fibrosis, Huntington's disease, and sickle cell anemia. Many such genetic disorders are easily identified through testing one's genetic makeup, or deoxyribonucleic acid (DNA). In many cases, although diseases may be detected early, symptoms cannot be prevented from emerging, and available treatments are modestly effective at best.

In rare cases, AD is due to a defective gene or mutation that is passed from a parent with the gene to one's child. Three such genes have been identified to cause AD.[5] This rare form of "familial AD," which affects probably less than 1 percent of all people with AD, is also unusual in that symptoms emerge in one's thirties, forties, or fifties. This form of the disease is sometimes referred to as "young-onset" or "early-onset" AD. The genes responsible for familial AD can be detected through blood tests and can actually predict if someone will become symptomatic. Genetic testing is recommended for families with a history of early-onset AD and should always be accompanied by expert genetic counseling. At present, physicians have no means of preventing the onset of symptoms after an AD gene has been identified. For example, a large family in the country of Colombia carries one such gene and is now part of a massive research study to determine how to reduce the risk of developing symptoms of the disease. In nearly all cases of AD, however, genes do not play a definitive role in the development of the disease, and therefore testing to identify a specific gene is pointless.

Although very few diseases pose a 100-percent risk of being transmitted from an affected parent to his or her children, a genetic susceptibility or vulnerability may be present in many, if not most diseases. In other words, genetics may play a partial role in the development of most diseases but rarely seems to play an absolutely causative role. Most chronic diseases, including AD, are likely caused by a complex interaction of genetic and environmental risk factors.

In some cases, a gene known as Apolipoprotein E4 variant (ApoE-4), has been identified that increases one's susceptibility or risk for developing AD late in one's sixties, seventies, or eighties. Again, a blood test is available to identify this susceptibility gene. However, because the influence of the ApoE-4 gene is much weaker than that of truly causative genes, being neither necessary nor sufficient for the development of AD, testing provides little useful information in most situations. Even people who test negative for the ApoE-4 gene can still be at increased risk, if they have an affected relative. To be clear: this gene and others that may be identified in the future do not cause AD but may increase one's risk of developing the disease late in life. Because the ApoE-4 gene has poor predictive value and no proven interventions to reduce the risk of AD yet exist, several organizations including the American College of Medical Genetics and the National Society of Genetic Counselors have recommended against testing for this susceptibility gene.[6] Nevertheless, some physicians may use this test to support other clinical findings in order to clarify a diagnosis of AD.

Advances in understanding human genetics may ultimately lead to ways of blocking the action of defective genes and promoting drugs that mimic genes with protective effects. In the meantime, the search continues for factors in the environment that put us at risk for certain diseases, including AD, so that we can modify our lifestyles and ward off these diseases. If reversible risk factors can be identified, we may discover clues about preventive measures and better treatments.

How Alzheimer's Disease Changes the Brain

Progressive severe loss of memory—routinely forgetting conversations or that one ate at a particular restaurant might be examples of this—and impaired thinking abilities are not a normal part of aging. Rather, such problems may be signs of dementia—a loss of brain functions due to an organic cause. *Dementia* is a generic term that includes a host of symptoms related to brain failure. Problems with concentrating, following directions, handling finances, and keeping track of conversations are all common symptoms of dementia. Just as we speak of many causes of conditions such as heart failure, kidney failure, or liver failure, brain failure also has many possible causes. And although dementia also can be traced to dozens of causes, AD is by far the leading one.

The human brain is at the core of our existence, but we take its functions for granted until disease or trauma disables it. Our brains enable us to think, remember, see, breathe, walk, talk, read, write, touch, taste, and perform countless other acts. Everyone's unique personality stems from a complex set of brain functions. Through the relatively new field of neuroscience, we are just beginning to understand the intricate workings of the brain and the disabling effects of brain diseases and brain injuries, such as concussions experienced by football players.

Essentially the brain is a high-powered communications network on a small scale—it weighs only 3 pounds, about 2 percent of total body weight. The brain has an amazing capacity to organize and execute complicated functions without any conscious effort on our part. The average human brain has an estimated 100 billion nerve cells, or neurons, that normally work in harmony through a series of intricate chemical signals to store, process, and retrieve information. There are thousands of potential connections, or synapses, for each of these 100 billion cells. Thus, the number of connections in the brain may total hundreds of trillions! Normal brain functions are threatened if a disease, such as AD, or injury disrupts cell-to-cell communication. AD destroys cells in the parts of the brain that control memory, as well as other key functions such as reasoning and language, and when nerve cells in the brain die, they are not replaced.

When the brain is working properly, it is as if a huge symphony orchestra is simultaneously creating, playing, and recording a stream of masterpieces. If a member of the orchestra misses a note, then the music changes slightly but imperceptibly. As the faltering musician misses more notes, the change in the quality of the music is noticeable only to someone with a highly trained ear. Other members of the orchestra may play louder or work harder to compensate for the faulty or missing notes. If yet another member of the orchestra loses track of her part, the change in the music becomes obvious to others. Other musicians may be thrown off by the discord, and they too may misplay their parts. Soon, the most skilled and hard-working musicians may no longer be able to keep pace with the challenges of the diminished orchestra. Eventually the entire audience will start to be bothered by the strange sounds emanating from the once-perfect orchestra. This model of an orchestra that falters musician by musician until musical chaos ensues is a good analogy for the process of a dementia like AD.

As the above noted continuum illustrates, AD unfolds over a period of many years. The slow damage to and death of nerve cells that accompanies the disease used to be visible only upon microscopic examination of certain regions of the brain. Recent advances in technology, however, now can detect such abnormal changes using brain scans and spinal fluid with increasing accuracy but are not yet perfected for everyday use by physicians. The disease typically occurs first in a thimble-sized area known as the hippocampus, believed to be the main recorder of new memories. It also attacks certain other areas, notably the cerebral cortex. AD is also characterized by reduced production of certain brain chemicals called neurotransmitters, which enable nerve cells to receive and send messages and help us to carry out innumerable functions, both intellectual and physical. When the brain no longer produces enough of these important chemicals, nerve cells can no longer communicate effectively, and they eventually deteriorate and die. Exactly how this process evolves in the brain is the subject of great speculation and controversy among researchers.

The nerve cells affected by AD are vital for memory and other so-called higher brain functions such as speaking, comprehending, reading, abstract thinking, and calculating. In particular, short-term memory, or the ability to remember recent events, is initially impaired by AD, but other brain functions may be affected at the same time. Moreover, nerve cells that control functions such as movement and vision may be well preserved. As a result, the physical appearance and bodily functions of a person with AD remain largely intact. The disease may be discerned only in the person's ability to remember, learn, and think.

In a sense, a person with AD loses the "glue" that enables new information to "stick" in the brain. This means, on the one hand, that if information is not sticking or being recorded properly, then new learning cannot take place as efficiently as it did in the past. On the other hand, information that is already firmly glued or recorded in the brain may continue to be retrieved from what is called long-term memory. This explains why someone with AD cannot remember a recent conversation but can reminisce in great detail about a childhood experience.

As mentioned earlier, AD does not occur suddenly, as if a switch that's been in the "on" position is suddenly turned "off." Damage to the brain may be so subtle at first that no one, including the person with AD, may notice that it is happening. Nerve cell death and chemical deficiencies may continue over a period of many years before symptoms become evident. The slow and insidious onset is similar to that commonly experienced by people with heart disease. It quietly takes its toll. Some people with AD develop a mild form of the disease in which symptoms slowly worsen for five or more years. Indeed, they may develop other life-threatening conditions before they need full-time care. Other people with AD decline rapidly to the point of total disability within just a few years. Reasons for these different rates of decline are still not clear.

It is clear, however, that having AD alone or in combination with other illnesses shortens life expectancy. Studies have differed in calculating how long a person will live, on average, after a diagnosis of AD. The general rule of thumb is that a person diagnosed with AD can expect to live half as along as a peer who does not have the disease. For example, a seventy-five-year-old woman today can expect to live another thirteen years. A seventy-five-year-old woman with AD, in contrast, can expect to live for six and one-half more years. Keep in mind that such estimates do not take into account a number of factors such as current health and lifestyle that could increase or decrease life expectancy.

AD has probably been around ever since human beings first managed to extend life beyond six or more decades, although relatively few people lived to an advanced age until the twentieth century. Over two thousand years ago, Plato declared that "a man under the influence of old age could not be responsible for his crimes." Writing in the second century, the Greek physician Galen theorized that a physical ailment might be responsible for the mental decline of some older persons. In centuries past, the symptoms now attributed to AD were referred to as insanity, senility, or hardening of the arteries.

Then, in 1906 a German physician named Alois Alzheimer published a now-famous case of a woman, Auguste Deter, who died at age fifty-five after her memory and other brain functions became progressively impaired over many years.[7] Upon her death, Dr. Alzheimer examined her brain under a microscope and found tiny abnormalities or lesions, now known as amyloid plaques and neurofibrillary tangles, throughout her gray matter. He attributed the impairments in her memory, thinking, language, and judgment to these physical changes throughout her brain. At that time, the symptoms that Dr. Alzheimer described were fairly common among older people. However, it was believed that these symptoms were a normal consequence of aging, and they were known as "senile dementia." After Dr. Alzheimer reported his findings to the medical community, the symptoms he described were classified as "pre-senile dementia of the Alzheimer's type," referring to the rare cases affecting middle-aged people. More than a century later, the case of Auguste Deter was re-examined with modern medical technologies, and it was discovered that she carried one of the rare genetic mutations responsible for AD.[8]

Finally, in the 1960s, scientists discovered a link between this unusual disease affecting a tiny number of middle-aged people and the common condition of "senility" observed among elderly people. Both age groups not only shared similar symptoms during their lifetime, but they also exhibited the same pathologic abnormalities or lesions in the brain. It was at this time that AD gradually became a subject of intense scientific inquiry. The story of how AD originates in the brain and manifests in behavior is still being written more than one hundred years after Dr. Alzheimer first described it. Yet even today basic questions about whether the plaques and tangles are causes or effects of the disease are not fully answered.

Research into most age-related conditions, including AD, is still relatively new, despite the fact that the older population in developed countries is growing like never before in human history. In fact, the age group older than eighty-five is the fastest-growing segment of

American society. AD is now estimated to affect more than five million Americans, the vast majority of whom are more than sixty-five years old. And nearly fourteen million Americans will have the disease by the year 2050, if means of prevention are not found.[9] The so-called age wave has resulted in scientific investigations into all aspects of aging. After decades of scientific neglect, the "little-known disease process" named for Dr. Alzheimer is finally getting the attention it rightly deserves. Yet in spite of major advances in understanding AD over the past thirty years, relatively little is known about its underlying causes, and as a result, it has been difficult to develop effective treatments. Means of prevention or a cure will remain elusive until answers to basic questions about its multiple causes are discovered.

Getting an Accurate Diagnosis

AD is by far the most common form of dementia, but many other types exist as well. Some can be reversed with proper treatment, but most, like AD, are irreversible. Table 1.1 lists some of the less-common types of dementia that sometimes mimic AD. The first purpose of a thorough medical evaluation is to distinguish between reversible and irreversible forms of brain failure. Receiving a proper diagnosis is the starting point for understanding troubling symptoms, causes, treatment, and prognosis.

Table 1.1. Other Reversible and Irreversible Dementias

Some Reversible Types	Some Irreversible Types
Metabolic disorders such as a thyroid gland problem or vitamin deficiency	Vascular dementia (tiny or big strokes)
Infections in the blood or spinal fluid	Lewy body disease
Major depression	Frontotemporal degeneration
Brain tumor	Primary progressive aphasia
Intoxication due to drugs or alcohol	Creutzfeldt-Jakob disease

With most diseases, simple blood or urine tests can help a physician to make a diagnosis. For example, a small blood sample can help a doctor readily detect if a person has diabetes. As noted above, however, no single, simple test currently exists to detect AD, which partially explains why most people with the disease are never officially evaluated or diagnosed. Tests involving blood, urine, skin, eye pupils, and sense of smell have been tested and thus far proven unreliable in identifying a definitive biological marker for AD. Researchers are making strides to identify a quick-and-easy method of detecting the disease using brain scans and spinal fluid. Such tests are being used at research centers, but nothing is yet available for use by physicians in an office setting.

A specific diagnostic test for AD would help doctors quickly rule out the disease or distinguish between AD and related disorders. It might also help prompt early intervention, when the benefits of treatment are likely to be greatest. Such a test may be on the horizon and will receive much public attention should it become available. Yet the symptoms of AD manifest in such a classic pattern that even without a single test, it is possible for an experienced physician to make an accurate diagnosis in the vast majority of cases and to differentiate it from less-common forms of dementia.

Perhaps the most important part of a diagnostic evaluation involves gathering information about the past and current symptoms. People showing signs of dementia may have varying degrees of insight into the nature and severity of their difficulties. Therefore, obtaining an accurate history about the symptoms from a knowledgeable informant is key to sorting out the medical facts. The observations of spouses, life partners, close relatives, and friends can be crucial in helping a physician make an accurate diagnosis.

Most types of dementia are progressive, and the manner in which symptoms unfold usually will support or rule out certain diagnoses. A process of eliminating other causes of dementia is the typical means of arriving at a probable diagnosis. This is done through blood tests to look for chemical excesses or deficiencies, and a brain scan to rule out a tumor, stroke, or other abnormality. These tests can be done on an outpatient basis, and most costs are covered by health insurance. Table 1.2 summarizes the tests used to detect and sort out the symptoms of dementia.

Table 1.2. The Most Common Diagnostic Tests for AD

Commonly Used	Sometimes Used
History and physical exam	Battery of psychological tests
Neurological exam	Spinal tap to check cerebrospinal fluid
Cognitive screening test	HIV blood test
Blood and urine tests	Brain biopsy
Brain scan (CT or MRI)	Brain scan (PET or SPECT)

In most cases, it is not difficult to make an accurate diagnosis of AD, despite the lack of a simple biological test. Unfortunately, because of the lack of a single foolproof test, some physicians overlook the disease or mistake it for a related condition. Identifying AD when it coexists with another condition can be difficult. For example, a person who is severely depressed may be forgetful in ways similar to a person with AD. Many reversible forms of dementia such as major depression, pernicious anemia, brain tumors, hypothyroidism, infections, and nutritional deficiencies may mimic the symptoms of AD, and many medications can induce memory impairment and other symptoms associated with the disease. A careful evaluation can yield the correct diagnosis, since the symptoms found in most cases of AD conform to a typical pattern. What is confounding is that AD is sometimes combined with other irreversible types of dementia such as Lewy body disease or vascular dementia.[10]

A physician will use a number of diagnostic tools to sort out the facts. First, rather simple mental-status tests enable a physician to assess memory, language, and organizational abilities, and screen for the presence of cognitive impairments. The most commonly used screening test is known as the "Mini-Mental State Exam" and involves a brief series of questions and tasks that identify the presence and severity of impairments.[11] Another simple test is known as the "Mini-Cog," in which a person is first asked to remember and a few minutes later repeat the names of three common objects and then must draw a face of a clock showing all twelve numbers in the right places and the time as specified.[12] Performance of everyday tasks, such as handling money or using a telephone, should also be explored through a separate interview with a reliable informant.

If memory loss or any other brain impairments are revealed, additional tests should be done. These include a physical and neurological examination, blood and urine tests, and a brain scan. Although such tests seldom show abnormalities, every possible explanation must be considered. In some cases, further laboratory tests, brain imaging tests, and a battery of psychological tests conducted by a specialist may be needed to clarify a diagnosis. However, a limitation of psychological tests is that they usually are geared to older people with average levels of education and intelligence and may not be sensitive enough to detect subtle abnormalities among those with high levels of education and intelligence. In such cases, close family members and friends can corroborate whether a decline in mental functioning has been detected. Therefore, detailed psychological tests may be useful but are not essential in making a diagnosis of AD.

As already noted, recent improvements in brain imaging techniques have made it possible to see changes in the living brain due to AD. However, examination of brain tissue under a microscope is currently the only accepted method of absolutely confirming the presence of AD. If a biopsy is performed, a small piece of brain tissue is removed surgically. Then an expert examines the tissue, looking for the tiny brain lesions (plaques and tangles) that would lead to a definitive diagnosis of AD. However, a brain biopsy is potentially dangerous, so it is very rarely done. The most common way of confirming a diagnosis of AD is through a brain autopsy—an examination of the person's brain that is done after his or her death. However, as stated above, a reliable diagnosis can be made without an expensive brain scan, a biopsy, or an autopsy based on a close scrutiny of the individual's symptoms. Using the established criteria, most physicians today are confident in making this "probable" diagnosis:

The Value of a Diagnosis

All physicians are familiar with AD, but not all of them are comfortable making the diagnosis. Some see the lack of a single accurate test as an impediment. Others may refrain from making the diagnosis because they think that the drugs that are currently available are not worthwhile. Current drug treatments are modestly effective at best in treating symptoms of the disease. Still other physicians mistakenly attribute the symptoms of the disease simply to old age, as if serious mental decline with aging is inevitable. And some physicians may error on the side of caution by labeling someone with the less-threatening condition now referred to as MCI. Many problems associated with AD are intertwined with the psychosocial issues of families caring for the person with the disease, and some physicians, mostly because of time constraints, do not get involved in these complicated matters. Unfortunately, health insurance does not adequately reimburse physicians for the time and effort to deal with this disease effectively. Even the most compassionate physician may not be able to address the array of challenges presented by AD.

Nevertheless, these considerations should not deter a physician from making a medical evaluation or from referring you and the person with symptoms to a specialist. He or she may need to be prompted to take the symptoms seriously, which means you may need to make a phone call to the physician's office before a visit, or you may want to engage the physician directly in a discussion about your observations. The changes you are seeing are troubling, and by any standard, it is reasonable to request a medical explanation. If indeed the condition is labeled MCI instead of AD, the symptoms represent a significant departure from one's past performance and adjustments need to be made in one's lifestyle. Assertiveness may be required on your part to elicit the physician's cooperation in completing a thorough medical evaluation and obtaining needed help.

Other good reasons for getting timely help are summarized below. If a physician cannot personally offer this measure of help, then he or she should refer you to others who can be of assistance.

Reasons for Obtaining a Diagnosis

- to rule out reversible forms of dementia
- to provide a context and explanation for symptoms (see Chapter 2)

- to obtain appropriate medical treatment (see Chapter 3)
- to consider whether or not to enroll someone with AD in a research study (see Chapter 4)
- to help you understand your changing roles and responsibilities (See Chapters 6 and 7)
- to ease communication among all concerned (see Chapter 8)
- to plan for the future (see Chapter 9)

The medical specialists most attuned to diagnosing AD are neurologists, psychiatrists, and geriatricians. Nevertheless, all physicians caring for older persons should be attentive to the warning signs of the disease and, in most cases, should be able to rule out reversible causes of dementia. Because of the uncertainty and implications of MCI, a specialist should probably be consulted to obtain the most detailed testing. And specialists should certainly be consulted in all unusual cases, particularly if the person exhibits symptoms affecting one's personality and behavior. If there is still uncertainty about the diagnosis after an expert opinion, a follow-up examination in six months may clarify the situation, since AD involves a progressive worsening of symptoms. Specialized diagnostic clinics can be found at all of the AD research centers in the United States funded by the National Institute on Aging (see the Resources in the back of this book). Many states also provide funding for "memory clinics" and other diagnostic centers. These centers and local chapters of the Alzheimer's Association in the United States or the Alzheimer Society in Canada can refer you to a specialty clinic or other known experts in your area.

Disclosing the Diagnosis

After tests have ruled out reversible causes of dementia and the established criteria for AD have been met as described above on page 12, the physician should sensitively explain the test results, diagnosis, and treatment options to the individual who has been tested, you, and any others close to the situation. The physician should also address questions regarding the potential causes of AD and the progression of the disease, and give recommendations regarding educational and supportive services.[13] Again, the problems associated with MCI should not be minimized, and its implications should be explained. Ample time should be available for questions and answers. People who are unable to attend this important meeting should be given the opportunity to join via videoconference or teleconference with the permission of the diagnosed person. For the sake of informing others unable to attend this meeting, audiotaping or videotaping should be allowed. Also with proper permission, you can also request a copy of the medical records for later review and distribution to other interested parties.

Family members and friends sometimes worry about the reactions of the person being given the diagnosis of AD. It may be useful for the physician to speak with you first, but this is not the suggested option. A separate meeting does allow time for your immediate emotional reactions and a discussion of the way in which the diagnosis will be presented to the individual with the disease. A fear commonly expressed is that the news will be devastating and depressing to the individual with the disease. These negative expectations are understandable in light of the grim stereotypes about AD. However, the person with the disease usually receives the diagnosis with little or no emotion and few if any questions. For the sake of unity in your relationship with the person with AD, therefore, it is better for everyone to meet with the physician at the same time so that the diagnosis and reactions can be shared.

Those with AD seldom grasp the full implications of the diagnosis. Even those who are well aware of their symptoms ordinarily do not appear overwhelmed by the news. It seems that the ability to understand the magnitude of the situation may be blunted by the disease itself. Those with AD typically do not share the same perceptions of the disease as others close to them. In a sense, the disease is often accompanied by a cushion that softens its meaning for the affected person. Most people with AD already know that something is not right with their memory and thinking. Putting a label on their symptoms may make no difference to them. However, receiving the diagnosis may eliminate their need to cover up or to try to compensate for their difficulties.

Some people with AD ask a few basic questions but usually defer to their family for clarification or further information. Still others admit to a memory problem but dismiss it as nothing unusual for an aging person. Some feel relieved that their symptoms can be attributed to a disease instead of something that they have failed to control with their willpower. After being given his diagnosis, one man commented, "I knew something was not right, so I have been working hard for quite a while to cover up the problem. Perhaps now I don't have to be so careful if others know what's going on with me." A woman with AD shared this desire for openness: "The fact that I have Alzheimer's is something I want everyone to know. I want people to be sincere in what they say to me, and I want them to know that I'm not contagious!"

Others are relieved because they can now discuss their difficulties openly for a change instead of feeling embarrassed by their need for help. They may want to plan out how to make the best use of their time before the disease disables them any further. Yet others may also wish to take part in a support group for persons with AD in order to obtain advice and information about coping with the disease. Appropriate reading materials suited to those with the disease are noted at the end of this chapter. Many people with AD exhibit little or no desire to further discuss their diagnosis and its implications, and they should not be pressed to do so.

The physician may opt to avoid using the term *Alzheimer's disease* out of respect for the family's expressed wishes. The more benign term, *mild cognitive impairment,* may seem useful, but it is misleading if indeed the symptoms fit the criteria for a diagnosis of AD. Vague or misleading terminology may sound comforting but detracts from the reality that significant changes are afoot. Years ago, physicians and families were reluctant to tell individuals about a diagnosis of cancer. It is now recognized that this deceptive practice created more problems than it solved. Openness and honesty have now replaced the conspiracy of silence that once prevailed in relation to disclosing the diagnosis of cancer. The same principle should apply in relation to telling an individual about his or her diagnosis of AD or the condition known as MCI.

Moreover, a central principle of medical ethics is each person's "right to know." Everyone has the legal right to access the private information contained in his or her medical records. Disclosing the diagnosis enables people with AD to participate fully in decisions about themselves both now and in the future. For example, the diagnosis must be given if the person with AD is to make an informed choice about participating in research studies. A diagnosis helps the person with AD and others to make legal and financial plans in an atmosphere of openness and true dialogue. The benefits of telling the truth about the diagnosis invariably outweigh the perceived benefits of secrecy. Even though a family may wish to shade the truth or avoid it altogether for its own reasons, this approach should be challenged. Nevertheless, since the family ultimately must live with the consequences of the diagnosis, each family's unique preference regarding disclosure of the diagnosis must be respected.

Although the hallmark of AD is loss of recent memory, many other possible symptoms are associated with the disease in its early stages. The next chapter focuses on the many symptoms that may be manifested in the early stages of Alzheimer's disease.

2 Symptoms of the Early Stages of Alzheimer's Disease

I know that I have a problem, but it doesn't bother me.
If you're going to have it handed to you, you have got to
take it, anyway. So that is the way I look at it.

Glenn Campbell, country music star,
diagnosed with Alzheimer's disease

Forgetfulness may be sporadic and seem insignificant in the early stages of both MCI and AD, but it becomes more persistent over time. It may take months or years before you, as a close relative or friend of someone experiencing gradual memory loss, begin to notice any pattern. A particularly troubling incident or a series of minor incidents may trigger an appointment for a medical evaluation. Although persistent memory impairment is the key feature of MCI and AD, subtle changes in one or more brain functions such as language, orientation, perception, and judgment may also be evident. In this chapter, I describe the many possible symptoms of the early stages of AD in terms of their impact on you and the person living with these symptoms.

The early stages of AD usually involve difficulty remembering recent episodes—such as forgetting an encounter with someone or losing or misplacing something. These instances gradually begin to disrupt one's customary lifestyle. The person experiencing memory loss may require regular reminders about tasks such as keeping appointments, cooking meals, or paying bills. At the same time, this same person may appear to think and behave normally much of the time.

However, this appearance of normalcy is deceptive, since microscopic damage to the brain is creating a host of practical difficulties. There may be valiant efforts to hide or compensate for such difficulties, but eventually, people close to the situation sense that something is not quite right. As the disease slowly advances, the need for help becomes more apparent. Therefore, it is important to understand the usual signs and symptoms of the disease, as well as many unusual features that may be manifested.

What Is Recent Memory?

The type of memory affected by AD is generally called "recent memory." A person whose recent memory is impaired typically forgets events that took place within the past hour, day, or week. Entire episodes or fragments of an episode cannot be recalled because new learning does not occur or is disrupted. Recent memory is quite different from remote memory, which involves events, places, or people from the distant past and often remains intact in the early stages of the disease. For example, a person with AD may not be able to recall what she had for breakfast today but may well recall the details of a high school prom some sixty years earlier. The ability to perform personal-care tasks such as dressing and bathing usually remains intact, too. Lots of abilities may be well preserved at this stage, whereas other abilities may be impaired. There is great variability among affected people in how the disease is first manifested and progresses over time, although impairment of recent memory is the common feature.

Beginning Signs

As noted in the first chapter, what are commonly referred to as the early signs of AD do not actually mark the beginning of the disease; rather, they are the first *observable* and persistent signs. At this point on the disease continuum, the threshold between MCI and AD has been crossed, although that turning point is largely a judgment call by a physician. Most family members of a person with AD are able to recall unusual incidents that occurred months or years before a loved one was diagnosed with AD. They may have dismissed these warning signs as nothing more than eccentric behavior or as a normal part of the aging process. Only when a pattern emerges over time are these strange incidents put into the proper perspective. The case of former President Ronald Reagan is typical in this regard.[1]

Although Mr. Reagan did not reveal that he had been diagnosed with AD until November 1994, his memory was undoubtedly declining for years before then. When asked if Mr. Reagan showed signs of the disease during his second term as president, which ended in January 1989, former White House physician Burton Lee told *USA Today*, "It was noticeable that there was something wrong there, but we figured it was just the natural aging process. Nancy was going to protect him, and she did. She kept him further and further out of the flow."[2] Likewise, Edmund Morris, Mr. Reagan's official biographer, provides many examples of changes in his memory and thinking in *Dutch: A Memoir of Ronald Reagan*.[3] To outward appearances, Mr. Reagan carried out his public life for many years without difficulty. For example, by all accounts he delivered a rousing speech at the Republican National Convention in 1992. Although Mr. Reagan still had the capacity to deliver a prepared speech, he likely could not recall its details a short time later. Such inconsistencies and a slow progression of symptoms are common in the early stages of AD. Mr. Reagan's earliest symptoms probably began to make sense to his family and friends after a pattern emerged and a diagnosis was obtained. Only in hindsight do episodes of forgetfulness that meant little when they occurred take on new meaning. This is the classic pattern of the disease in its early stages.

It is easy for casual observers to overlook the disease in its early stages. Even keen observers may be initially fooled by the consistent symptoms. Since we have no single objective test for diagnosing AD, physicians may be hesitant to make the diagnosis. And the decline in memory often associated with aging, including MCI, confuses the situation. For example, allowances are made for an eighty-year-old person who is a bit forgetful because of the common belief that some degree of memory loss is to be expected at that advanced age. But if the same level of memory loss were observed in a fifty-year-old person, there would be cause for alarm. In other words, societal expectations often come into play in distinguishing between normal and abnormal forgetfulness.

People with AD naturally follow a pattern of compensating for their deficits, keeping them hidden from others as long as possible. They may deliberately avoid situations that challenge their faulty memory, such as having to remember names at a social gathering. After all, it is only human to want to avoid embarrassment and to be at one's best in everyday situations. They may quietly retire from their jobs, for instance, after realizing that work demands are becoming too challenging. Once they retire, others may not readily notice their deficits because they no longer have the intellectual demands of a job. At home, they may gradually turn over certain responsibilities to others, such as balancing a checkbook, shopping for food, or preparing income taxes. They may avoid new and unfamiliar places and people, and rely on stock phrases and old memories in conversations instead of revealing their inability to keep track of new details. Usually, these are not deliberate attempts to cover up but, rather, they are unconscious efforts to adapt to changes in memory and thinking. Often their spouses and others close to the situation unwittingly adapt to these changes and slowly assume a more active role in the relationship.

Loved ones usually notice a significant problem once the affected person becomes taxed beyond his or her mental abilities. While daily routines may not reveal much, stressful episodes may bring symptoms of the disease into the open. For example, the drastic change in lifestyle required as a result of a spouse's death is enough to uncover symptoms. In addition to the loss, the spouse can no longer help in taking care of the details of everyday life. In one case, a son describes how he first became aware that there was a serious problem with his mother after his father's sudden death: "I knew Mom was slipping a bit, but Dad rarely complained. He gradually took over most of the household tasks. After he died, Mom seemed really confused. She not only missed him on an emotional level but on a very practical level too. I had no idea of how forgetful she was until he was gone."

Any major change in the routine of an affected person may be sufficient to bring out the symptoms of AD. For example, when a person with AD goes on vacation, he or she may experience confusion and may even get lost. One woman traced her first awareness of her husband's AD to their trip to Europe:

First, he did not participate as usual in the planning of the vacation. He seemed anxious while packing his bags. He had trouble remembering the location of hotels as well as our itinerary. He seemed really out of sorts at times, but then he would seem okay at other times. He was fine when we got back home, but later I began to notice little things that made me suspicious all over again.

An Emerging Pattern

One's abilities to store, prioritize, and recall new information are brain functions that slowly break down with the onset of AD. At first, family members usually write off these memory lapses as absent-mindedness or a lack of attention. Forgetfulness may be easily overlooked as part of the human experience. After all, there are so many minute details to remember that the brain naturally filters out trivia. However, these incidents eventually become part of a disturbing pattern, indicating AD.

In the early stages, the affected person may be able to remember certain trivial details while forgetting matters of great importance, or vice-versa. Loved ones may rationalize these memory lapses as random blips when, in fact, they may be initial signs of the disease. In some cases, the person with AD is the first to notice the problem and to complain about changes in memory and thinking.

Forgetfulness in the early stages of AD may take a variety of forms. At first, it is mild and erratic. Those affected forget things more often than they did in the past. They may forget appointments, parts of conversations, or even entire conversations. Even when reminded, they may forget again just minutes later. They may even forget that they have forgotten! Or they may repeat the same statements or questions over and over. Their attempts to compensate by writing out reminders eventually prove inadequate as the problem worsens. Their written notes may actually add to their confusion. They may forget about appointments in spite of reminders offered by other people. They may forget to pay bills, or they may pay the same ones more than once. They may forget that they have food cooking on the stove and end up with burned meals. Learning and remembering new information becomes a real problem.

The person with AD typically has good days and bad days or good moments and bad moments within a given day. He or she may remember some things and forget others within the same hour. Ann Davidson writes in her memoir, *Alzheimer's, A Love Story: One Year in My Husband's Journey*:

> Julian can't remember that his underpants are in the dresser, yet he usually remembers to come home on time. He doesn't know the location of the wall plugs when he tries to vacuum, yet he knows how to go alone to the library. He's capable in some areas, impaired in others. His abilities fluctuate day-to-day, maddeningly inconsistent.[4]

Such ups and downs in one's functioning may prevent other people from putting together the pieces of the puzzle. There is also a natural tendency to deny the reality that a loved one's growing problems may be due to an irreversible disease. Family members and friends may act as if no difficulties exist or minimize their importance so that the situation ultimately resembles the proverbial "elephant in the living room" that everyone tries to ignore. Sometimes a crisis has to occur before others awaken to the fact that something is not right: the person gets lost while driving, utilities are cut off due to nonpayment of bills, a house fire results from food forgotten on the stove. In some instances, it may take an "outsider" to recognize that the seemingly disconnected incidents are part of a medical problem such as AD. The following excerpts are taken from conversations with family members who were asked to recount their initial awareness of a loved one's memory problem.

George described how he first became aware of his wife's memory problem about four years before she was diagnosed with AD at age seventy-six:

She was having a problem with remembering names that I thought was excessive, even for an older person. I could not accept that this was simply the natural aging process. When she was interviewed by our family physician, he said there was no problem whatsoever and that she was perfectly normal in every aspect. In turn, I accepted the medical opinion and did nothing at all about it for quite some time.

Paul looked back to a year before his wife's diagnosis of AD at age sixty-two:

It seems like during the course of that year she was becoming constantly forgetful of things, like misplacing her glasses and car keys. Any time she needed something, she would write and staple notes around her purse handle. Sometimes she would have fifteen or twenty notes stapled there. I really took notice when I looked for the pills that she was supposed to take every day for her thyroid condition. It turned out that the bottle had been empty for a couple of months. When I asked her if she had discontinued the pills, she said that she had just forgotten. Around the same time, she also stepped down from her position at work because she said it was getting to be too much for her worsening memory.

Because of a family history of the disease, Lucy explained that she became aware of signs of it in her mother about three years before she was diagnosed at age seventy-seven:

We noticed my mother started to forget little things. We've had experience with this before. My mother's sister succumbed to Alzheimer's and my mother's father also lived to the very late stage of Alzheimer's. The forgetfulness was becoming more commonplace—simple things like where she put things around the house. I noticed another classic sign in the repetitiveness. We also noticed a drastic change in her personality over the past year—she wasn't as outgoing or adventurous as she used to be. So we had her evaluated by a neurologist who confirmed what we had suspected from the start.

Robert recalled a particular event that triggered his awareness of his mother's loss of recent memory:

The first time I noticed a real problem was after her hysterectomy, when she was recovering in the hospital. They wanted to train her to get around and use the washroom at home. She was horrified that she couldn't remember what her bathroom looked like at home, but she remembered what the bathroom looked like in a house that she lived in when she grew up, maybe sixty years earlier. She could see the past very clearly in her mind, but she couldn't remember the present. She thought she was going crazy. That was when I figured out there was something up. I could see that her mind at that point was very fragile, and that the sedation and other medications had set this off. She was never the same thereafter. I know I began to keep a closer eye on her after that hospitalization.

Mike lived a thousand miles away from his eighty-year-old widowed mother and saw her just twice a year. He reflected on her beginning symptoms, six months before her diagnosis:

On the phone she seemed just fine, but when I visited her she repeated questions quite often and reminisced about the past more than usual. I discovered that she had not paid a few of her bills, but she gave some excuse that led me to believe that it was a mere oversight. When these things were happening, I was not alarmed at first, but my suspicions grew over time.

Dorothy recalled the time she first noticed her mother's memory loss, about eighteen months before her diagnosis: "She would ask questions that I assumed she knew the answers to. She began to repeat herself, especially asking the same question that had been answered just a short time ago. I thought it was due to her aging."

Eleanor noted the change in her husband about five years before he was diagnosed at age eighty:

We were with a group of friends, playing really simple card games, and he decided he did not want to play anymore. He said the games were stupid. Even then I suspected that he was just saying that because he could no longer remember the rules. He had always had an excellent memory, but when he began to routinely forget appointments, I knew something was not right. My initial reaction was to insist that he make a greater effort to remember. I am afraid I put him through a miserable time.

As the above examples indicate, family members are usually puzzled by the difficulties that they notice in their loved one for some time before they realize that a disease may be in progress. Most people do not initially act on their feeling that something may be wrong, or they deny the severity of the problem. Fear and stigma associated with AD are real impediments to seeking out a diagnosis. Waiting for a couple of years before seeking out a medical explanation is common.[5]

Other Troubling Symptoms

Other symptoms may appear simultaneously with the impairment of recent memory, or they may develop over time. In most cases, although these other symptoms may be the first signs of AD, the central problem of memory loss doesn't lag far behind. These difficulties are generally mild in the early stages but clearly represent a departure from the individual's previous level of intellectual functioning or behavior. The following list summarizes common symptoms in the early stages of AD:

Always present
- impairment of recent memory

One or more sometimes present
- difficulty with reasoning
- disorientation
- difficulty with language
- poor concentration
- difficulty with spatial relations
- poor judgment

Noncognitive or behavioral changes sometimes present
- personality changes

- delusional thinking
- changes in sexuality
- diminished coordination
- diminished or lost sense of smell

One or More Symptoms Sometimes Present

In addition to persistent loss of recent memory, one or more common symptoms of AD will sometimes be present in the early stages. These include occasional or regular difficulties with reasoning, orientation, language, concentration, spatial relations, and judgment. The appearance of such symptoms over time varies from person to person but all of them usually become prominent as the disease advances. At first, however, these difficulties tend to be mild in nature.

Difficulty with Reasoning

Reasoning, or the ability to think logically, is often the second area beyond memory that is affected by AD. This impairment typically affects the person's ability to understand or solve practical problems. Like other symptoms in the early stages of AD, this symptom comes and goes at first. The affected person may become disconcerted if faced with a task involving a series of steps, such as handling money, doing calculations, cooking a meal, driving a car, or using household appliances and tools. Gloria explained that her husband had always been handy around the house but was stumped one day when faced with a relatively simple task:

> The first time I really began to notice there was a problem was one day when he tried to install a screen in the door. He stood there with the screen in his hand, looking at the frame and said to me, "I can't figure out how to do this." Then I began to reflect on other things that hadn't seemed right. I recalled that months earlier he had also said it was getting hard to balance the checkbook and had asked me to figure it out. He had always done the bills. These difficulties he was having were inconsistent, so I think we had been easing into things. When he said, "I can't do this" or "I can't figure that out," I realized that I wasn't just imagining things.

A problem with reasoning was described by Alex who reported that his wife had always been adept at managing their household expenses but began to make errors:

> When she began to forget to buy certain items at the grocery store, I did not think much about it. But when I discovered that some bills were not being paid and that the checkbook was a mess, it was a clear signal that something was not right. When I brought the problem to her attention, she tried to downplay the fact that changes were afoot. I kept a close eye on things from then on.

Disorientation

Confusion about time and space is fairly common in the early stages. The person with AD may get mixed up about directions and become lost or may not know the current day, month, or even year. Bill recounted the first sign of changes in his wife's ability to navigate their community:

> I noticed it in her driving at first. She had lived in our town all her life and always knew how to get around the area. One day she had to go to the bank and then to the insurance office. However, she had to come home after going to the bank because she didn't know how to get to the insurance company. She was also unable to keep track of her purse and was misplacing things. Her missing purse had become kind of a joke for the past four years. I think I just kind of grew accustomed to it, not necessarily thinking that it was Alzheimer's.

A woman with AD in the early stages describes her warped sense of time:

> Time means nothing to me. I rarely know the day of the week or the date. This bothers me a lot, but we have worked it out. George just says, "You have an hour before we go, so start getting ready." Since time is not there for me, I nap in my chair sometimes and when I awaken, I panic because I can't understand why I'm alone in the house—even though it's a work day for George. I'll dash around the house looking for George, or I'd have this awful feeling that I'm babysitting and can't find the children.

Difficulty with Language

In the early stages of AD, affected people don't have as much difficulty with the *mechanics* of speech as they do with the *rules* of speech that make verbal communication effective. They might have trouble finding the right words or remembering names. Even common objects like a shoe may be forgotten or misnamed as a sock. Their ability to process information may be slowed, resulting in long pauses or lapses in concentration during conversation. The overall richness of their vocabulary may diminish and so may the ability to articulate thoughts and feelings and to comprehend the speech of others. (See Chapter 8 for more information about communication difficulties and for suggestions on dealing with them.)

The first changes Winnie noticed in her husband were in his language ability:

> It was not so much his memory as his speech. Some of his sentences would be backward. He would mix up the sequence of the words. I was getting frustrated, and so I made an appointment with a neurologist, thinking that perhaps he had a mini-stroke or something. He was examined, but all the tests were normal at first. Another year passed before his doctor agreed that his memory problem had progressed and his coordination had started to diminish a bit. Only then did the doctor say he had Alzheimer's.

Poor Concentration

A person's ability to concentrate or to pay attention may diminish in the early stages of AD. This difficulty may manifest itself in reading with little or no comprehension or in being unable to follow a conversation. An individual may respond more slowly than usual to everyday situations. Richard noted his wife's growing difficulty holding a conversation:

> Sometimes she'll be talking and there will be a lapse in the conversation, and she [will] say, "Oops! The train left the track! What were we talking about?" I think it is more than forgetfulness. Sometimes she cannot pay attention. She seems to be easily distracted by other signs and sounds that compete with her brain.

Joan commented on her father's diminished concentration:

He used to be able to stay focused on reading a book or doing a chore around the house. He could occupy himself for long periods of time, but now his attention span is very short. It's disconcerting to see this change in him.

Difficulty with Visual Perception and Spatial Relations

The human eye depends on the brain to organize and interpret what is being seen. Judging distances and recognizing familiar people or objects are sometimes difficult for a person in the early stages of AD. In effect, the brain distorts visual images. This phenomenon, known as "agnosia," is an unusual first symptom in the early stages of AD that may appear later on. The following stories by two spouses highlight how difficulty with visual perception and spatial relations heralds additional symptoms.

John recalled that his father was the first to notice changes occurring in his visual perception:

He said he was tripping on stairs because he was having difficulty determining the space between them. It was as if the stairs were running together. He also complained that words appeared jumbled on printed pages. He would see things from afar and grossly misjudge their appearance. Of course, we thought it was his eyes at first, but the ophthalmologist said his eyes were fine. A short time later, the memory problem emerged. Again, he was the first one to notice this, too!

Don described his wife's early symptoms as difficulty with judging distances while driving, with other symptoms following:

About three years ago she was involved in a car accident on a road that was wide enough for eight trucks to go through, and yet she hit a parked car. I sensed that something wasn't normal when she had a couple more fender benders. After that, there wasn't really anything until last spring when I noticed she was forgetful, leaving purses, not taking messages, and she was not as neat with her appearance. Nothing drastic, but something was different. Also, people who didn't see her frequently would ask me what was wrong with her. They said she wasn't the same person—she wasn't outgoing or fluid with her speech and movement and thinking. I think it was the fact that other people were telling me that my wife had changed that made me aware of the fact that she was having these problems.

Poor Judgment

Making sound decisions depends on memory to an extent, but it also requires logic and reasoning. Distortions in the thought process may lead a person with AD to make inappropriate decisions. For example, a man in the early stages of AD impulsively bought an expensive new car, even though he could not afford it. Another man was scammed by a telemarketer, much to the chagrin of his daughter who noticed unusual charges on his credit card bill. In another case, a woman gave away most of her life savings to an unscrupulous neighbor. Another woman with AD turned up the thermostat in her home to eighty-five degrees, and the intense heat nearly killed her. Such bad choices usually represent a radical departure from one's previous habits and should be viewed as a potentially dangerous symptom of AD.

Noncognitive or Behavioral Changes

In addition to the intellectual impairments described above, certain other symptoms may be present from time to time or regularly. These include a range of personality changes, delusions, and changes in sexuality, physical coordination, and the sense of smell.[6] Again, not everyone with the disease has these symptoms. They tend to appear occasionally in the early stages, and become more common in the later stages of the disease, but the frequency and severity of these symptoms vary from person to person.

Personality Changes

Personality changes are seldom dramatic in the early stages of AD. However, the person may not seem like his or her "old self" in some ways. The most notable change is usually diminished drive or lack of initiative. People who are normally active may become passive, assertive people may start deferring to others. People in the early stages of AD may show a lack of interest in people and activities that they previously enjoyed, such as family gatherings, social events, and hobbies. This growing sense of apathy or loss of initiative can be puzzling. Such changes in mood and behavior are often misinterpreted as symptoms of depression. Although symptoms of AD and depression can occur together, generally speaking a loss of initiative may be due solely to AD and may be unresponsive to treatment with antidepressants. Luke recounted the change in his wife after they had relocated to a new home:

> She had a complete change in her personality once we got there. She normally was outgoing and curious, but she became a recluse. She wouldn't go anywhere without me. After a while, the confusion and memory problems set in.

Some people with AD may become self-centered and ignore the feelings of others. Such insensitivity may be offensive to others unless it is correctly interpreted as a sign of the disease. Judy initially worried that her marriage was falling apart because of the change in her husband's personality:

> He no longer seemed interested in me, which was quite out of character for him. He became increasingly self-absorbed, to the point that I thought he didn't care about me, or anybody else for that matter. I was beginning to believe that our marriage was on the rocks for the first time in forty-nine years.

Some people with AD may become less inhibited in their speech and behavior. Someone who may have been calm and patient in the past may now seem short-tempered. Likewise, someone known to be passive and quiet may become opinionated and outspoken. Impulses previously held in check may no longer be fully controlled. For example, a daughter complained that her mother, who had AD, had always been "prim and proper" but had developed a pattern of expressing herself in an offensive way: "My mother never used foul language in the past, but now she is doing it freely with no hint of embarrassment.

She can swear a blue streak now, which can be quite embarrassing. It's almost comical at times."

Sometimes people with AD may express a surprising degree of irritability or even outright aggression toward others, especially loved ones. Such disturbing behaviors typically stem from their feeling fatigued, overwhelmed, or frustrated. It is important for you to remember that verbal and physical outbursts are symptoms of the disease and should not be interpreted as personal attacks. There is almost always an underlying cause that triggers these unpleasant occurrences. To the person with AD, hostile remarks and acts may be means of self-defense in response to situations that they perceive as threatening or confusing. It may take some detective work on your part to figure out what triggers the antisocial behavior and how to minimize it or prevent it from happening again.

Delusional Thinking

Delusions refer to false, fixed beliefs. In AD they usually take the form of allegations, such as of infidelity, financial exploitation, and similar personal offenses against others close to the affected person. Delusional thinking is actually rare in the early stages of AD, and it is typically coupled with the loss of recent memory. Delusions may appear so irrational and out of character that they stir family members to seek a medical explanation. Peter noted that his wife became convinced that he was having an extramarital affair, in spite of all evidence to the contrary:

> She began to accuse me of infidelity—for the first time in fifty-two years of marriage! She claimed that whenever I left her alone I was seeing another woman. It was completely absurd, but she became wildly jealous and suspicious. All my efforts to reassure did not help. Only later did I understand this behavior as a symptom of her disease.

In another case, Joan's mother-in-law accused her of stealing some of her clothing:

> It was preposterous to think that I would be interested in her clothes. She apparently misplaced some of her things and decided

to blame me for some strange reason. She was convinced that I was at fault. At first, I made the mistake of trying to reason with her. Her continuing accusations really strained our relationship for a while. I learned not to argue with her.

Changes in Sexuality

Healthy sexuality depends on a variety of complex physical and psychological factors related to the brain, and changes in sexual function may be common in the early stages of AD. Diminished sex drive is probably the biggest issue. Men may have difficulty attaining or maintaining an erection, while women may experience lack of vaginal lubrication. Whether these problems are related to disruption in brain pathways affecting sexual arousal or are rooted in emotional reactions to other brain changes due to AD is not well understood. Maria described her husband's sexual difficulties:

> He wanted to have sex, but he was unable to sustain an erection. After a while he gave up trying, and I thought it was perhaps my fault. That was about the same time I first noticed his memory problem.

George noted that his wife lost all interest in sex:

> We had a good sexual relationship, but she lost her desire. I would make advances but she would turn me away. I did not know why until someone explained that this change in her might be due to her disease. The explanation was helpful in reducing my frustration with her lack of interest.

Sexual interest may actually sometimes increase in the early stages of the disease. Josephine explained the change in her husband's sex drive:

> We had always enjoyed a close, loving relationship, but he became even more amorous after he suddenly retired. I later found out that his retirement was linked to his declining job performance. Shortly thereafter, I began to notice his problems with memory and thinking. Although his brain was failing, his sexual appetite was growing!

Because of embarrassment, many affected people unfortunately never address these sexual changes. Marriages may suffer over this sensitive matter, and spouses may retreat from each other or get into conflict. Partners of those with AD should recognize that changes in sexual functioning are not necessarily a sign of problems in the relationship. Rather, a diminished or heightened sex drive should be seen within the context of other symptoms associated with AD and should be discussed openly.

Diminished Coordination

Although most physical functions are typically unchanged in the early stages, sometimes a person with AD may walk cautiously or more slowly than usual, or have difficulty with getting up from a chair or out of bed. Some studies have shown that diminished coordination and walking as well as falls and stumbles may actually herald the onset of AD before memory loss is evident. Some people may also experience minor difficulty with complex and fine motor functions involving eye-hand coordination and rapid hand movements, which may be manifested in illegible handwriting or trouble using utensils or tools. This motor impairment may also get in the way of driving a car safely. How AD damages certain nerves and muscles while leaving most of the affected person's physical abilities intact is not yet understood. Medications, arthritis, and other medical issues may cause coordination problems, so these possibilities need to be ruled out by one's physician.

Lost Sense of Smell

Strong evidence suggests that people with AD tend to lose their sense of smell.[7] Just like the brain interprets what the eyes see, the brain interprets what the nose smells. Damage in different parts of the brain will affect different senses. This particular sensory deficit, also known as "olfactory dysfunction," can be caused by many other medical factors apart from AD. This problem has some practical implications that require monitoring. For example, someone may not be able to smell burning food or a gas leak in one's home. A lost sense of smell should be seen as another potential symptom of AD.

Take Action

The early stages of AD are characterized primarily by loss of recent memory but may be accompanied by other symptoms. Loved ones may notice these subtle changes, but they are easy to miss. As the disease slowly advances, seemingly disconnected incidents of forgetfulness and other warning signs begin to form a troubling picture. You and others who are close to the person with AD should acknowledge these changes and recognize that a medical problem is probably unfolding. A proper diagnosis, treatment, and planning are indicated for the sake of all concerned.

An experienced physician is the best person to sort out the various pieces of the puzzle and help you with the next steps. Your job at this juncture is to make sure that the physician knows about all of the symptoms and conducts a thorough evaluation. It will be helpful to write down exactly what happened that led you to suspect something was not right and to share this history with the physician. Your observations as well as observations by other people will be useful in making a diagnosis.

A final thought is necessary about obtaining a diagnosis, and it relates to another symptom: lack of awareness. Relatively few people with AD are fully aware of their problems, so few will seek a diagnosis on their own. In most cases, people are brought to the attention of their physicians at the behest of their concerned relatives or friends. And some of these people with symptoms are completely unaware that they are experiencing any problem whatsoever. For these people, it is more than denial, which can be considered a normal coping response to their symptoms. Rather, they are oblivious to their symptoms due to a biological problem: The part of the brain responsible for personal awareness is apparently damaged in such cases. They may seem unconcerned about problems that are readily apparent to other people. How then does one get such a person to agree to a medical evaluation?

It is recommended that a call be placed to the person's physician in advance of a routine medical visit to share one's observations so the physician can further investigate. If possible you should accompany the person to the physician's office. You could ask to be allowed to be part of the examination and interview. Medicare now pays for annual "wellness visits," and a check of one's memory is supposed to be done. The Alzheimer's Association has recommended simple screening tools that physicians and other health-care providers may use to test one's memory.[8] Screening should lead to additional tests to finally set the record straight. Once a diagnosis of AD has been made, questions turn to medical treatment. The latest available information about treatment and current trends in research are addressed in Chapter 3.

3 The Treatment and Prevention of Alzheimer's Disease

*Every complex problem has a solution
that is simple, neat, and wrong.*

• • • H. L. Mencken

In this chapter I will review current options for treating AD as well as some options that may become available in the future for treating, slowing down, and preventing the disease. At present nothing is available to stop or reverse symptoms. A handful of drug treatments are available that are modestly effective in improving symptoms and slowing down the progression of AD, but these do not work in all cases. Better drugs may be on the horizon. These include drugs that are in testing phases at research centers and clinics, mainly in North America, Europe, and Japan. And although claims that certain herbs and dietary supplements may enhance memory have not yet been substantiated, some alternative medicines may also prove beneficial. I caution a healthy skepticism about anything that claims to be helpful but lacks solid scientific evidence. After all, more than one hundred drugs that were tested for AD over the past decade actually failed to yield positive results. The chance of a dramatic breakthrough any time soon is slim, so you must beware of hype.

It seems that the media report on a new study about AD every month. However, most of these studies have no immediate applicability to people with the disease. Lots of these news reports are studies that took place with cells or animals in a research laboratory. For example, despite important new research on the brain's ability to regenerate cells and a potential vaccine for AD, it remains to be seen if these findings yield any real benefits for people with the disease. The results of other studies involving a small number of people may be tantalizing but may not prove useful in larger studies. Likewise, advances in gene therapy and cell transplantation for diseases affecting the brain have no relevance for people with AD in the near future. Therefore, we should be careful about reading too much into preliminary reports. Although researchers are making progress in the treatment of AD, the pace thus far has been very slow due to the mysterious nature of the disease. Increased government funding is urgently needed to better understand the origins of the disease; that is the only way to develop truly effective treatments or means of prevention.

Currently no drugs exist that benefit everyone with AD. Just four drugs have received approval from the Food and Drug Administration (FDA) of the U.S. government. These drugs are modestly beneficial for less than half the people in the early and middle stages of AD. Although their benefits are usually short-lived, some evidence suggests that they may also have longer-lasting effects. Because there is no way to predict who may benefit from these drugs, every individual with AD should probably try one of these drugs on a trial basis to determine its effectiveness for him or her. As with all other drugs, they should be taken under the supervision of an experienced physician who can help you in assessing the safety and effectiveness of the treatment. However, you may be the best judge to observe any benefits or side effects.

Most drugs tested for AD so far have not targeted the underlying pathology of the disease described earlier, including amyloid plaques and tangles. Such drugs are currently being developed. Instead, drugs tested and approved to date have attempted to replace chemicals that are deficient in the brains of people with AD. This approach follows the one used in treating Parkinson's disease, another common brain disorder that results in slowed movements, rigidity, and tremors. Deficiency of a chemical called dopamine is chiefly responsible for the symptoms of Parkinson's. There are several prescription drugs available that attempt to compensate for this chemical deficiency, and, as a result, people with Parkinson's disease often experience temporary relief of symptoms. The problem with a single-drug approach to treating AD is that people with the disease have a whole host of deficiencies in their brains, and currently no single drug is capable of replenishing all of these chemicals. It is generally accepted that replacing deficient chemicals and treating symptoms alone is not the best approach for treating AD. Treating and preventing roots causes of the disease is the current trend, but progress is painstakingly slow.

Current Treatments

So far, as noted, after rigorous testing over a period of many years, only four drugs have been approved by the FDA for treating AD. These drugs are available only through a written prescription. Other drugs are in various phases of testing in the United States and elsewhere, and their entry into the marketplace is expected in the next few years.

Table 3.1. Medications for Treating Alzheimer's Disease*

Table 3.1 lists the four drugs, the stages of the disease they are intended for, their recommended daily dosages, and how these drugs are administered.

Brand Name (generic)	Drug Class	Stage of AD for which FDA has Approved	Typical Daily Dosages	Administration
Aricept (donepezil)	Cholinesterase inhibitor	Early, middle, late	5, 10 or 23 mg	5 mg/day and can be increased to 10 mg/day after 4–6 weeks. After 3 months, can be increased to 23 mg/day.
Exelon (rivastigmine)	Cholinesterase inhibitor	Early, middle	6–12 mg	One 3 mg, 4.5 mg, or 6 mg capsule twice daily in the morning and evening with food; also available in liquid form.
Exelon Patch			4.6, 9.5 or 13.3 mg	Apply one patch once daily to the upper or lower back, upper arm, or chest.
Namenda (memantine)	NMDA receptor agonist	Middle, late	20 mg	One 10 mg tablet twice daily, morning and evening, with or without food; also available in liquid form.

(cont'd.)

Table 3.1. Medications for Treating Alzheimer's Disease* (cont'd.)

Brand Name (generic)	Drug Class	Stage of AD for which FDA has Approved	Typical Daily Dosages	Administration
Razadyne (galanta-mine)	Cholinesterase inhibitor	Early, middle	16–24 mg	One 8 mg or 12 mg tablet twice daily (morning and evening with food); also available in liquid form.
Razadyne ER (Extended Release)				One 16 mg or 24 mg capsule in the morning with food.

* This chart is current as of 2013; for the latest prices on many of these drugs, go to www.drugstore.com.

Aricept, Exelon, Razadyne, and Namenda (see Figure 3.1) passed strict testing standards and showed through independent studies that they improved memory and thinking abilities and increased overall functioning. Namenda stands out because it is the only one of these drugs that is not approved for use in the early stages of the disease and works on a different chemical system than the other drugs. As a result, it is sometimes prescribed in combination with one of the other drugs, even in the early stages. All the drugs potentially slow the progression of AD but do not change the underlying pathology of the disease. Curing, reversing, or stopping the course of the disease is a goal but is not yet possible.

Cholinesterase Inhibitors

Aricept, Exelon, and Razadyne are in a class of drugs known as cholinesterase inhibitors. Aricept is the most widely prescribed drug in this class. All of these drugs block the brain enzyme cholinesterase that normally clears up excess amounts of a key brain chemical known as acetylcholine that is essential to memory, learning, and other functions. This class of drugs essentially aims to artificially mimic a process that occurs naturally in the brain. Evidence indicates that all of these drugs have modest but meaningful effects on about half of those in the early stages of AD. Benefits include slight improvement for a period of up to a year or more in memory, language skills, and ability to handle tasks like personal grooming. These drugs may help to slow one's expected rate of decline.[1] Thus, these drugs potentially prolong one's independence for a longer period of time than expected without their use. In effect, they may be equivalent to "turning back the clock" in the typical disease process.

Aricept, Exelon, and Razadyne differ slightly in their chemical makeup and how they affect one's brain chemicals. As a result, people who do not benefit from one drug may benefit from another one. Likewise, people who cannot tolerate side effects of one drug may do well with another one. There is some evidence that if one drug is not effective or is not well tolerated, switching to another one might be beneficial. The bottom line here is to keep an open mind about trying different drugs. Again, not everyone responds favorably to these drugs, so expectations should be tempered.

No study has shown added benefits of taking two of these drugs together and the risk of serious side effects may increase when two or more of these drugs are taken together. Benefits reported for all of these drugs tend to occur at higher doses, which also increases the likelihood of known side effects such as diarrhea, vomiting, and nausea. And as with any type of drug, careful monitoring is required with all of the cholinesterase inhibitors. Due to their potential for slowing the progression of AD, these drugs also have been tested to see if they might delay the onset of the disease among people with mild cognitive impairment (MCI), but results thus far have not been favorable. Nevertheless these drugs are sometimes prescribed off-label for people with MCI in an effort to improve symptoms and stave off AD.

Namenda (Memantine)

Namenda, known also by the generic name memantine, is the second most widely prescribed drug for AD. It is listed by itself in a different class because it blocks excess amounts of glutamate, another brain chemical that is important for learning and memory. This drug was available for many years in Europe before it was approved for use in the United States for people in the middle to late stages of AD.[2] Namenda can be used by itself, but some evidence supports the benefits of combining Namenda with Aricept, Exelon, or Razadyne.[3] However, people in the early stage of AD are generally started with one of the latter drugs. Although the FDA has not approved Namenda for treating people with early-stage AD, physicians may choose to prescribe it off-label. The only way to determine which drug or combination is better for a particular person is simply trial and error. It is important to keep an open mind during the process to determine what works or what works best.

What are the practical benefits of all of these drugs? Again, it appears that about half of the people in the early stages of AD who take them respond favorably, at least for a while, in terms of symptomatic improvement or stability (not getting worse). Improvements in memory, thinking, and concentration are the most frequently reported positive changes. Family members report that the diagnosed person often seems "sharper" or more attentive during drug treatment. The person's ability to recall recent events and to complete personal care and household tasks may also improve. Problems such as repeating questions, misplacing objects, or becoming confused in new surroundings may be eased. Also, one's overall mood and behavior may be improved. Although the changes are seldom dramatic, the families of those with AD are usually grateful when any improvement is observed. No change in the typical progression of the disease is considered beneficial, too. On the other hand, some people with AD remain stable without using these drugs. Because the rate of progression varies from person to person, it is sometimes difficult to gauge if stability is due to a drug or to the slow course of the disease in any given person. Because it is tempting to look for improvement even where none exists, the true effectiveness of a particular drug should be evaluated after it has been tried for a few months.

One practical consideration is the cost of these drugs: They are expensive. Without insurance, they cost $150–200 per month. Medicare—the U.S. health-insurance program for people age sixty-five and older plus younger people who qualify for Social Security Disability—will pay for these drugs if you have enrolled in either a Medicare Prescription Drug Plan (Part D) or a Medicare Advantage Plan (Part

C). For details, contact Medicare at (800) 633-4227 or go to www .medicare.gov. For people who are enrolled in the combined federal–state program known as Medicaid, these drugs are covered. For details about how to reenroll in your respective state, go to http://medicaid .gov. Some states also have established drug assistance programs for citizens who are not poor but meet other qualifications.

For those who do not qualify for the above programs and cannot afford to pay for drugs, these states and the drug companies have set up assistance programs so that the drugs may be received free or at reduced cost. The Partnership for Prescription Assistance is an organization that serves as a single point of access to more than 475 public and private programs that help qualifying people without prescription drug coverage get the medicines they need free or nearly free. Call (888) 477-2669 or go to www.pprax.org.

Medical Foods

A number of supplements and products called "medical foods" purporting to improve memory and thinking skills are likely to be on the market in the near future. Big food companies see opportunities for making huge profits by selling medical foods. In general, to be considered a medical food, a product must, at a minimum, meet the following criteria: The product must be a food for oral or tube feeding; the product must be labeled for the dietary management of a specific medical disorder, disease, or condition for which there are distinctive nutritional requirements; and the product must be intended to be used under medical supervision. Unlike drugs, medical foods and the more-common supplements are not allowed to claim they help cure illnesses, but they are often used in conjunction with drugs to treat a disease. Although medical foods are subject to the general food-and-safety labeling requirements set forth by the FDA, they do not have to be approved by the FDA and undergo much-less-stringent testing than drugs that must demonstrate both safety and effectiveness. Some manufacturers require a physician's prescription to use medical foods, but not always. Because medical foods are not drugs, insurance coverage may vary considerably.

One such food already on the market for AD is Axona, a combination of compounds naturally found in the diet but not usually together. Alzheimer's is thought to hinder the brain's ability to break down glucose. According to Axona's marketing materials, the food supplement provides an alternative energy source that the brain can use instead of glucose. Axona is a powder to be mixed with water or other foods/liquids to be taken by mouth once a day, preferably at breakfast or lunch. It is administered under physician supervision and dispensed by prescription. Relatively small studies of people in the early and middle stages of AD who took Axona showed some improvement in cognitive function.[4] Another medical food, Souvenaid, is also a patented combination of nutrients in powdered form to be mixed into a drink or milkshake. Souvenaid is already available in some European countries and Australia, and the giant food company behind the product is hoping to bring it to the United States after further research is conducted. Preliminary studies have shown potential benefits for people in the early stages of AD.[5] Thus far, the Alzheimer's Association has avoided endorsing the use of medical foods for AD in light of the lack of rigorous scientific data to substantiate their effectiveness.

Progress in Treatment

At any given time, several dozen drugs for AD are in various phases of testing at research centers throughout the world. It may take several years before the value of these experimental drugs is fully understood. All of them are attempts to improve upon the performance of the drugs already approved by the FDA. In the coming years, we should hope to see a number of additional drugs offering more meaningful and longer-lasting benefits to people with AD. Clearly, a vaccine to treat or prevent AD would represent a quantum leap forward in medicine. However, attempts to develop a vaccine thus far have failed.

Many other interventions are being tested to slow down the progression of AD. For example, a current government-sponsored study at many sites throughout the United States employs a pacemaker-like device that is surgically implanted into brains of people in the early stages of AD. The device, which provides deep-brain stimulation and has been used in thousands of people with Parkinson's disease, is seen as a possible means of boosting memory and reversing cognitive decline. This study marks a new direction in clinical research designed to slow or halt the disease. Even existing drugs used for other medical conditions are being attempted to treat AD. For example, a low dose of insulin sprayed into the nose has shown promise in preliminary studies among people with AD.

Drugs, medical devices, and medical foods differ from more common and even more lightly regulated supplements, or "nutriceuticals." Health-food and vitamin stores are big business, but their products are not subject to much more than safety testing. Claims about potential medical benefits are not based on solid scientific evidence. Some manufacturers have been sued by the U.S. government because of false or misleading claims. Two large-scale studies of gingko biloba, widely used and marketed as a memory-boosting supplement, offer a useful lesson in exercising caution about supplements. Researchers studied the use of this supplement among thousands of volunteers in the United States and France, and results showed that gingko biloba had no effect in boosting memory or preventing AD.[6] Other substances supposedly can slow down AD but lack close scientific scrutiny. For example, coconut oil is being promoted as a treatment for AD, but there is scant science to support its use.

Research suggests that the death of brain cells occurring in people with AD partially results from the increased production of "free radicals," oxygen molecules that cause damage throughout the body. The potential benefits of antioxidants in slowing down and preventing this damage have been a topic of much speculation. With respect to memory, many preliminary studies involving animals and people have shown the benefits of foods loaded with antioxidants, such as spinach, blueberries, and strawberries. Whether such findings can be replicated in larger studies of people remains to be seen. Studies of other antioxidants—including supplemental folate, selenium, vitamin B-6, and vitamin B-12—have failed to show that the rate of decline can be slowed among people with AD. A growing number of studies have shown that older people who regularly got ample amounts of vitamin E or C through food but not supplements, lowered their risk of developing AD. These nutrients are naturally found in green, leafy vegetables but are also available as nutritional supplements in over-the-counter products. However, supplements have no proven benefits at this time.

The so-called Mediterranean diet has shown promise in promoting both heart health and brain health. This diet is inspired by the traditional dietary patterns of southern Italy, Greece, and Spain. The principal aspects of this diet include high consumption of olive oil, unrefined cereals, legumes, fruits and vegetables, as well as moderate consumption of dairy products, fish, and wine and low consumption of meat and meat products. Whether this diet can slow down the progression of AD or cut one's risk of developing AD is unproven.

Hormones

A hormone is a chemical released by a cell or a gland in one part of the body that sends out messages that affect cells in other parts of the organism. In essence, it is a chemical messenger that transports a signal from one cell to another. A number of compounds, both natural and synthetic, have hormonelike effects on humans that can change the body in the same way that hormones within the body do. There are more than fifty synthetic hormones available today for treating a variety of health conditions. For example, synthetic "human" insulin is now manufactured for widespread clinical use for treating diabetes. There are also hormones that supposedly slow the aging process and reduce the risk of Alzheimer's or slow its progress. None of these claims have been proven. Hormones such as estrogen, testosterone, melatonin, and progesterone may be useful for other medical conditions but lack solid science to support their use in treating AD.

Because no major medical treatments for AD yet exist and because the pace of research is slow, many people seek help outside the scientific mainstream. More and more people have become disillusioned about the limits of modern medicine in treating a variety of conditions and illnesses. Ancient practices such as acupuncture, acupressure, massage, aromatherapy, and herbal medicine have become increasingly popular. Billions of dollars are spent annually in the United States on alternative therapies. Many practitioners of complementary and alternative medicine claim to offer help and healing to people with medical conditions that are unresponsive to conventional treatments. Perhaps scientists will some day prove that some of these unorthodox therapies actually work. The interest in alternative medicine is bound to grow with the aging of the baby boom generation. The National Center for Complementary and Alternative Medicine, under the auspices of the National Institutes of Health, is charged with investigating these old and new forms of treatment. Call (888) 644-6226 or go to http://nccam.nih.gov.

The makers of dietary supplements and herbal remedies claim their products may improve memory or increase thinking and other brain functions. Garlic, ginseng, kava, green tea, and a host of others have been touted as memory enhancers or as natural means to improve one's concentration. These products can be sold in the United States without meeting the stringent guidelines the FDA sets for drugs, as long as the sellers do not claim to treat, cure, or prevent disease. Their popularity and huge sales indicate a widespread belief that these forms of alternative medicine must have some advantages. Thus far, however, no controlled studies have either proved or disproved claims of effectiveness for any of these products, and consumers may not have reliable information about their safety, effectiveness, or potency.

Among other claims, a natural product known as huperzine—an extract derived from a Chinese club-moss plant that is a traditional Chinese herbal remedy for fever—is supposed to enhance memory and concentration. Huperzine has similar chemical properties to the current class of cholinesterase inhibitors that are approved in the United States, and these claims seem to have some scientific basis, as evidenced in preliminary studies on rats and humans. Because huperzine is considered a dietary supplement and therefore is not within the realm of FDA regulation, it is available over-the-counter in nutrition stores throughout the United States. However, it probably deserves the kind of monitoring normally reserved for prescription drugs, according to some experts. The results of research studies on the effectiveness of huperzine in treating AD have been mixed, and the U.S. government-funded study proved disappointing.[7]

Although the desire to try out the vast array of available alternative treatments is understandable, it is also important to retain a healthy skepticism about unproven pills, procedures, and practices. Many well-meaning people believe that they have stumbled on a break-through without the benefit of rigorous methods to test their claims. Likewise, many unscrupulous opportunists are eager to prey on the vulnerability of people who are desperate for anything of potential value. If you are interested in pursuing alternative therapies, I recommend that you do so with a "buyer beware" mentality. In pinning your hopes on a quick fix for AD, you run the risk of both disappointment and exploitation.

The "Use-It-or-Lose-It" Approach

Questions often arise about the value of mental and physical exercises in preventing brain diseases or in increasing "brain power." This use-it-or-lose-it theory is gaining increased attention in scientific circles. Brain researchers are now finding that nerve cells in mammals' brains continue to generate long after maturation, suggesting that similar cell generation is probable in humans. Moreover, scientists are beginning to explore the effects of impoverished versus enriched environments on the brain. There is a growing consensus among medical research-ers that lack of mental or physical stimulation reduces the number of brain cells, whereas increased stimulation promotes the growth of new brain cells. Preliminary studies have shown that mental and physical exercise may play a role in delaying or preventing AD.[8] Intellectual exercises such as playing cards or chess, reading a book, taking a class, or attending a lecture or museum are both interesting and pleasurable, whether or not they ward off AD or slow its progression. The health benefits of physical exercise for the cardiovascular system are well documented and may well apply to the brain, too. Growing evidence suggests that whatever is good for the heart is probably good for the brain, too.

Recent years have seen an explosion of interest in improving mem-ory and concentration through computer programs and games and other learning protocols involving math and reading. Although these commercially available products are primarily marketed to people without AD, they are now being tested among people with MCI and the early stages of AD. Although memory training or brain exercises have not been proven to benefit people with AD thus far, such mental exercises can actually be counterproductive, since pressure to remember things may trigger frustration and lower an affected person's self-esteem. However, different types of stimulation have been shown to affect the mood and behavior of people with AD. For example, a loud and overstimulating environment can be agitating, while soothing music is known to have a calming effect on people with the disease. Ideas concerning suitable mental and physical activities for people in the early stages of AD are addressed in Chapter 10.

Participating in Clinical Drug Trials and Other Studies

Any new drug intended to treat people ultimately has to be tested on people in clinical trials, which determine if it is safe and effective, at what doses it works best, and what side effects it has. Standards for effectiveness and safety differ in each country. The FDA in the United States is perhaps the most stringent regulatory agency of any government in the world. Its goal is to ensure that all drugs meet the highest standards for safety and effectiveness through different phases of clinical testing.

Someone with AD may want to consider enrolling in one of the many drug trials being conducted at different places in the United States, or in other types of research studies. An obvious and legitimate reason for participating is self-interest. Most studies offer no direct or immediate benefits while others hold promise for a scientific breakthrough. Participation in research may also provide opportunities to become better educated about AD, to discuss ways of coping, and to feel supported by the professionals conducting the studies. Such benefits may be of interest to the person with AD and his or her loved ones.

The research that is often of most interest to people with AD and their families concerns experimental drugs. If the current AD treatments you have encountered prove disappointing, then your loved one may wish to enroll in a study of a newer, experimental drug. This may offer you reassurance that everything possible is being tried. The early stage of the disease is the proper time to consider this option, since people in later stages are typically excluded from participation for a variety of medical, legal, and ethical reasons. Even people in the early stages of AD may be excluded from participation due to strict criteria necessary to conduct proper testing. For example, someone who has other major health problems may not be eligible to take part in a clinical drug trial.

It is important to clearly understand the possible risks and benefits of participating in clinical drug trials. These risks and benefits must be fully explained in writing before your loved one with AD volunteers to enroll as a participant. An "Informed Consent" form should be read carefully and signed by both you and the person with AD. Participation in these studies involves no financial cost, and the risk of harm is usually minimal. All studies of experimental drugs are carried out at reputable research clinics located in universities, at medical centers, and within the community that are supposed to abide by the highest ethical standards and protocols. Table 3.3 lists the major reasons why participating in clinical drug trials may or may not be for you or your loved one.

Table 3.3. The Pros and Cons of Participating in Clinical Drug Trials

Pros	Cons
Free diagnostic tests and monitoring of memory, thinking, and other cognitive skills	Numerous tests, which can be tedious and tiring
Payment for travel costs to and time at the clinic	Many time-consuming appointments, which can be inconvenient
Access to experts involved in the study who can educate and support you	Potential side effects (e.g., nausea, insomnia, anxiety, etc.)
Possibility to be among the first patients to try a promising drug	Possibility of receiving a placebo (dummy pill) instead of the active drug
Chance to contribute to scientific effort to know what works and does not work	Chance of no benefit

It should be noted that participating in research is not for everyone. It boils down to a personal choice for those directly involved. Studies involve risks that may not seem worthwhile to you or your loved one.

One man with AD noted, "I don't like those stressful memory tests. Unless I can be guaranteed I will not get a placebo, an experimental drug is not for me." Time and energy are needed to participate, too. And there may be no real medical benefits. In fact, as mentioned, hundreds of drugs that have been tested for AD have failed, and only four have been approved despite the efforts of thousands of volunteers and the millions of dollars spent. It is important to be hopeful, but expectations should be set low for real breakthroughs. An altruistic outlook is helpful, too. For example, after taking part in a six-month study involving a new drug, one woman with AD remarked, "It did not work, but my husband and I were comforted knowing that we had done our part to answer the question about the drug's effectiveness. Besides, we got lots of attention from a fine group of professionals during the study."

To find out about research studies being conducted in your local area, contact one of the federally funded centers listed in the Resources section or go to the U.S. government website: http://clinicaltrials.gov. People with AD, their families, and others can also be matched to studies at www.alz.org/TrialMatch.

Clinical trials of new drugs are conducted in several phases over a period of many years, usually under the auspices of a pharmaceutical company but sometimes with the backing of government funding. Table 3.4 summarizes the phases of drug testing in the United States.

Table 3.4. Phases of Testing New Drugs in Humans

	Phase One	Phase Two	Phase Three
Typical Number of Participants	20–100 healthy volunteers	Up to several hundred volunteers at risk or diagnosed with AD	Up to several thousand volunteers at risk or diagnosed with AD
Length of Time	Up to one year	Up to two years	One to four years
Purpose	Mainly safety	Mainly effectiveness and a determination of dosage levels	Safety, effectiveness, and ease of administration

A promising drug is first tested for effectiveness and safety using test-tube and animal studies in the laboratory. This preliminary phase may last from one to six years, and if the drug shows enough promise, it moves to the first phase of human testing. This step requires the approval of the FDA. In phase one of human testing, the drug is tested mainly for safety among a small number of people, usually fewer than one hundred healthy volunteers; this phase typically lasts about a year. If the first round is successful, the testing moves to phase two.

In phase two, the drug is tested among several hundred individuals who have the disease the drug is intended to treat; this phase can last up to two years. In this phase, researchers employ a method known as a double-blind, placebo-controlled study. Participants are randomly assigned to two groups: One group is given the experimental drug, and the other group receives a placebo, which is a pill without active ingredients. The studies are considered double-blind because neither the participants nor the researchers know who is receiving the drug and who is receiving the placebo until after the study has been completed. A third party keeps track of this information to monitor any serious side effects of the drug and to complete an analysis of test results. If phase two is successful, then the next round of clinical trials involves an even greater number of people with the disease, from several hundred to a thousand.

In phase three, the double-blind, placebo-controlled method is again used. This phase may last from one to four years. During phase three, researchers may offer an "open-label" option as an incentive to participate in the study. In an open-label study, all participants who complete the study are given the option of taking the experimental drug for six months to one year before the drug manufacturer applies to the FDA for approval. If the drug proves beneficial and safe by the end of this third phase, then an application is submitted to the FDA for review.

Further testing may be required before the FDA makes a final determination to either approve or deny the new drug application. After careful scrutiny of all information regarding safety and effectiveness collected at all phases of testing, the FDA makes a determination whether the drug should be approved for public use, usually through a doctor's prescription. Even if a drug is approved, the pharmaceutical company is required to continue submitting reports describing the drug's performance. The approval process from beginning to end usually takes more than ten years and costs millions of dollars. The high price of new drugs is directly related to the research and development phases.

Much research focuses more on finding answers to basic questions about the nature of the disease than on drugs to treat it. There are studies to identify additional risk factors for AD, different methods of diagnosis, and nonmedical ways of treating mood and behavioral problems, to name but a few. Such research projects may not offer any immediate or personal benefits, but they may lead to knowledge that has practical applications for others in the future. Altruism is at the heart of participation in this type of research, and people with AD and their families often feel good about their roles as volunteers in this important work. Regardless of outcome, they know that they have done their share to expand knowledge about AD. They are like the builders of the European cathedrals that took decades to complete: Although they may never witness the fruits of their contribution, they believe that the combined efforts of many people will some day result in solving the great puzzle of AD.

Toward Prevention

The four drugs approved for the treatment of AD are modestly effective in slowing down progression for some people for a limited duration. Attempts to improve upon them have failed miserably over the past decade. The common understanding today is that all of these drugs have not made a significant difference because they have not been introduced early enough; even by the disease's early stages people's brains may be too damaged for drugs to be truly effective in all cases. Much attention is now shifting to treating or preventing the disease before full-blown symptoms actually appear—in the MCI and pre-clinical stages.

Given the intense interest in preventing or slowing down the progression of AD, what is really known from a scientific point of view? To separate fact from myth, the National Institutes of Health, an agency of the U.S. government, convened a panel of fifteen independent medical scientists in 2010.[9] This expert group carefully examined all published studies on nearly everything proposed to prevent the disease: physical and mental exercises, diet, social engagement, nutritional supplements, as well as anti-inflammatory drugs and drugs to lower cholesterol and blood pressure. They included an array of research about traits that might hasten the onset of AD, such as not having much of an education or being a loner. The panel rated scientific evidence as high, moderate, or low, depending on how confident they were in the findings.

Despite a wealth of studies, the panel generally judged that most studies conducted to date had limited data and that the quality of scientific evidence was low. Low confidence meant the evidence was so faulty that there was no way of deciding if a particular measure worked. The panel concluded that there was poor evidence, for example, that keeping your brain active, physical exercise, or eating a Mediterranean diet or foods rich with omega-3 fatty acids has a protective effect. Most studies assigned a low confidence rating had observed people who happened to use or not use a possible preventive measure and then determined whether they developed AD or not. Such studies, known as observational ones, are not the gold standard, like those in which people are randomly assigned to take a pill or do something like exercise, or not. Observational studies are useful in generating hypotheses, but they are not proof. If several well-done studies of this type come to the same conclusion, they can be valuable evidence. The panel found moderate evidence, not totally convincing but not worthless, for possibly reducing the risk of AD with the three FDA-approved cholinesterase inhibitors and vitamin E found in foods. The panel said it was highly confident in the findings for just one thing: Ginkgo biloba did not prevent AD. This negative finding was disappointing, to say the least.

In the end, the panel of experts unfortunately concluded that there is no persuasive evidence to date that AD can be prevented. Still, the panel noted, "We recognize that a large amount of promising research is under way; these efforts need to be increased and added to by new understandings and innovations."

Three research studies aimed at AD prevention begun in 2013 are worth noting: two studies involving drugs and another one involving physical exercise.[10] In all of these studies, the status of memory and thinking skills as well as AD-related pathology in the brain will be measured through cognitive testing, cerebrospinal fluid biomarkers, and brain imaging. Many years of careful study will be needed to draw conclusions about each study's merits. The first study, a $100 million project funded by a consortium including the National Institutes of Health, drug manufacturers, and private donors, is being conducted among people in their thirties and forties who have inherited one of the genetic mutations that eventually results in AD. The individuals to be tested are unfortunately destined to develop the disease but do not yet have its symptoms. Participants in this study will include 300 people in Columbia, South America (the site, mentioned earlier, where members of a large, extended family develop symptoms of the disease in middle age), and as many as 150 Americans who are AD "mutation carriers." These people will receive one of two experimental drugs that hold promise for clearing amyloid plaques, a hallmark feature of AD in the brain. Each drug has passed earlier clinical trials that evaluated safety and effectiveness. The awkwardly named drugs, crenezumab and gantenerumab, are already being tested among people with AD in several countries. Whether or not they have "preemptive" effects on those at certain risk of developing AD is a huge yet worthwhile gamble.

The second prevention study is targeting one thousand people ages seventy to eighty-five whose brain scans show amyloid plaque buildup but who do not yet have any symptoms of AD. They will get monthly infusions of the drug known as solanezumab or a placebo (dummy drug) for three years. Two previous studies of solanezumab suggested it might modestly slow decline in people in the early stages of AD.

The third prevention study, also funded by the National Institutes of Health, involves a supervised aerobic exercise program among people with MCI to determine if the typical progression to AD can be stopped or slowed. Physical exercise is widely recommended to maintain physical function and reduce risk of a number of age-related medical conditions such as cardiovascular disease and diabetes. However, exercise has not been shown in long-term studies to improve memory or alter brain pathology associated with AD. A consortium of more than seventy research centers around the United States, known as the Alzheimer's Disease Cooperative Study, is responsible for carrying out this five-year study.

Although the chance of dramatic progress being made in the treatment or prevention of AD cannot be discounted, smaller or gradual advances are more likely. Hope lies in numerous types of research studies being conducted by scientists throughout the world, especially in the United States. The speed at which treatment and prevention efforts are developed is generally related to the level of funding for research. Private funding of AD research has risen significantly in recent years. Yet sadly, federal funding of AD research in the United States remains relatively low compared to other major diseases, despite the enormous economic and human cost of the disease. As a result, progress is relatively slow. Advocates of an accelerated research initiative must push this agenda forward with public officials while continuing to raise funds for privately backed research efforts. Another way to get involved directly in such efforts is to participate as a volunteer in research programs.

The Limits of Medicine

As scientists work hard to put together millions of pieces in the AD puzzle, you should not feel compelled to spend precious time and energy looking for a remedy that has eluded countless others. The media regularly report new advances in AD research—most of these report preliminary findings may or may not have applications in the future. For now, understanding the symptoms, diagnosis, treatments, and research agenda is a good starting point for families and friends of those with AD. Accurate and updated information about the disease can be gleaned from a variety of sources—books, newsletters, scientific journals, and, of course, the Internet. And yet, knowledge about the medical aspects of AD reveals little about how to best care for someone with the disease.

Renowned physician William Osler, MD, once gave sage advice to physicians and medical students about their main priority: "Care more for the individual patient than for the special features of the disease."[11] Richard Taylor, forced to retire from teaching as a result of AD, shared a similar idea in his memoir, *Alzheimer's from the Inside Out*: "From my perspective as a person living with this diagnosis, there is far too much emphasis on the label, the name, and the symptoms generally associated with the disease and too little emphasis on the individuals who actually have the disease."[12] Medical science and professional health-care providers have relatively little to offer right now in the way of treatment and prevention, but there is a lot you can offer in terms of care. Human compassion, skill, and imagination may be far more effective than any drug to help someone diagnosed with AD. In the next chapter, I will focus on maintaining and enhancing quality of life through such nonmedical means.

4 A Good Quality of Life

Do whatever your ingenuity and your heart suggest.
There is little or no hope of any recovery in memory.
But a man does not consist of memory alone. He has
feelings, will, sensibilities, moral being...and it is here
that you find ways to touch him. In the realm of the
individual, there may be much that you can do.

A. R. Luria (Russian neuropsychologist)

The above quote by one of the leading brain scientists of the twentieth century addresses the stark reality that there is no way to restore brain cells after they have been destroyed by AD. And drugs currently available to treat the disease offer symptomatic relief but do not arrest or reverse the disease. The complex causes of AD remain mysterious. In the face of the limits of modern medicine, it is easy to become discouraged and to turn to unconventional and unproven ways to stop or slow the progression of AD. Countless hours and money have been spent searching for an elusive cure. I firmly believe that you should instead devote your efforts to finding ways to provide a good life for the person with AD. The above quote looks beyond biology and medicine to consider how to treat the person with AD in other ways to maintain and enhance one's quality of life. This is the great challenge for family, friends, and others involved in the life of someone with AD. It requires a team of caring, dedicated people.

It is common to think in terms of waging a war against a disease, such as the campaign that led to the dramatic discovery of a vaccine that has nearly wiped out polio worldwide. Similar language has been used to fuel funding for research into cures for other diseases like cancer, heart disease, diabetes, and AIDS. While no one discounts this line of thinking for AD, what can an individual and family do in the meantime? I suggest that it is useful to shift from the traditional medical approach focused on cure, rehabilitation, and symptom relief to maximizing quality of life as the primary goal of care. Rather than make someone better, the question becomes: How do we enhance one's strengths and abilities despite the disabling illness? This shift in thinking is no easy task in a culture where quick solutions to problems are expected. Rather than wage a war against AD, this new goal requires learning how to adapt to it. It also means confronting our own fears about losing memory, thinking, and other precious abilities.

For good reasons, AD has become the most feared disease in our society today. The disease makes a person exceptionally dependent on others, which is a state that runs counter to the Western values of individualism and personal autonomy. Nobody wants to fail at doing simple things for oneself. Nobody wishes to be a burden. Nobody wants to lose control of thinking and behavior. These are common fears about AD confronted by everyone involved in the life of someone who has been diagnosed. These fears may have been shaped by past personal experiences or by friends who have dealt with the disease. Many people have heard stories about those diagnosed with AD becoming aggressive or paranoid. Popular books, television, film, radio, the Web, and print media have also instilled fear by portraying AD as a "loss of self" or a "never-ending funeral" or "descent into madness." With such dire and disturbing images, it is no wonder that the thought of having AD strikes abject terror.

We have grown accustomed to expecting AD to play out as the worst of the worst diseases. In *Forget Memory,* Anne Basting criticizes prevailing stereotypes and points in another direction: "The stories we tell about dementia in the mainstream media create the backdrop against which we forge our understanding of and attitudes toward it." Basting argues that these fears, stereotypes, and stigma make the experience of AD worse for all concerned. Rather than wallowing in such a pessimistic and self-fulfilling prophecy, what if AD were seen as an invitation to accommodate a form of disability? What if hope for a good life replaced fear of a ruined life as the dominant way of thinking about AD? In spite of all the changes imposed by this disease, is a good life even possible?

Answers to such questions may seem beyond your imagination if caught in the medical approach to AD. Try to consider an alternative view. It may open your mind to new possibilities and the capacity to live with "a new normal." Olivia Ames Hoblitzelle chronicles her own adaptive approach after she suffered the "arrow of shock" when her husband was diagnosed with AD in her inspiring memoir, *Ten Thousand Joys and Ten Thousand Sorrows: A Couple's Journey Through Alzheimer's*: "Hob and I discovered perspectives and attitudes that lightened the burdens of illness. Determined to live the experience consciously and lovingly, we regarded this—the final challenge of our relationship—as an opportunity for openness to the unknown for learning, and above all, for deepening in love."[1]

What Is a Good Life?

Determinants of a good life are subjective, for the most part. There are indeed objective elements too, such as physical and mental health, the environment, and relationships. One may argue that basics such as food, shelter, and clothing are essential for a good life. Yet preferences for these things vary from person to person. Some people living in rundown shacks may feel happy, whereas some of those living in opulent mansions may be miserable. Someone in the early stages of AD may be angry, while another person in the advanced stages of the disease may be content. How a person appraises his or her overall life is a critically important factor. Ultimately, each person is the final judge of all of the factors to assess the quality of one's life.

A growing body of social research in the past decade has shed light on the issue of quality of life among persons with AD. Several surveys and methods have been developed to assess quality of life from the perspective of both diagnosed individuals and their families. People with AD have been asked to numerically rate their relationships with friends and family, physical health, energy, memory, living situation, mood, ability to have fun, and overall life quality. Likewise, their closest family members are asked to rate their loved one with AD on the same items. A consistent finding is that people with AD rate their own quality of life significantly higher than ratings assigned to them by their family members. There are several possible explanations for this difference. Perhaps people with AD adapt to their condition more readily than their families. They may see their cup as "half full," whereas families see the same cup as "half empty." People with AD may also find greater enjoyment now in the simple things relative to their past life. Family members may not have caught up to this positive change, or they may feel burdened by their own increased responsibilities. Regardless of the explanation, it is comforting to know that people with AD generally have a better life than others might imagine. This notion defies the stereotype that people with AD suffer a poor quality of life due to their limitations.

Although quality of life is highly subjective, conditions beyond mere survival are needed to experience a good life. In the past generation, a movement to consider health and wellness as more than the absence of illness has taken hold. The National Wellness Institute, the principal organization for wellness education, training, and research in the United States, defines the wellness concept as six dimensional. Figure 4.1 on the next page shows six dimensions commonly associated with personal well-being: emotional, intellectual, physical, social, spiritual, and vocational. A wellness approach to AD aims beyond the intellectual dimension that is often the central focus of AD.

Emotional Wellness: This dimension reflects the degree to which an individual feels positive and enthusiastic about his or her self and life. It concerns feelings of personal security and safety. It involves the capacity to manage feelings and behaviors, self-acceptance, and coping with stress and life's challenges. It also involves the ability to give and receive love as well as the ability to understand and express emotions.

Intellectual Wellness: This dimension concerns the complex abilities of one's brain to think, recall, create, communicate, and solve problems. It involves one's capacity to make good personal choices and enjoy meaningful activities on one's own terms.

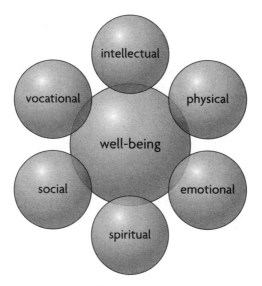

FIGURE 4.1 Six dimensions of life commonly associated with well-being

Physical Wellness: This dimension concerns physical health, fitness, and participation in personal activities for endurance, strength, balance, and flexibility. This concerns healthy lifestyle habits like a nutritious diet and regular exercise.

Social Wellness: This dimension concerns creating and maintaining healthy personal relationships. It concerns feeling comfortable and interdependent with others. It involves feeling connected to people, whether on a one-to-one basis or in groups.

Spiritual Wellness: This dimension is about seeking meaning and purpose in human existence. It concerns an appreciation for the depth and expanse of life and natural forces that exist in the universe. It involves feeling connected to someone or something beyond oneself.

Vocational Wellness: This dimension is about achieving positive personal and occupational goals and interests. It is linked to discovering one's "calling" in life and sharing personal talents. It means feeling good about one's contributions to others and the world. It is not necessarily tied to a job or employment status but to one's role.

To consider the importance of any of these dimensions of wellness, imagine a man named Fred, a forty-eight-year-old crane operator who was severely injured in a car accident, resulting in paralysis in both of his legs. Such a blow to Fred's physical well-being can be expected to affect other dimensions of his well-being, particularly if his personal identity was strongly tied to his physically demanding job. He must now use a wheelchair and rely on others, and he can no longer enjoy the same level of independence he had prior to the accident. His emotional well-being may be upset. Fred may fall prey to anger and depression, or he may be able to work through his feelings of loss to a renewed sense of himself. His relationships with his wife and children may be threatened, too, but his disability might also enable the family to draw closer together. He may lose easy access to his other relatives and friends or find new ways of connecting with them. Fred's spiritual well-being may be affected as he calls into question why God allowed this to happen to him. A spiritual crisis may result in turning away from or drawing closer to his God and his religious faith.

Fred may no longer be able to work or work in the same capacity, but accommodations may be possible. If there was a chance he could work again, an employer might make accommodations both in the nature of a job and in the workplace. Society has made all sorts of accommodations for disabled people in the past generation, especially those with physical disabilities. If Fred is unable to work again, he presumably would be eligible for disability payments through government or private insurance. No stigma would be attached to receiving these benefits. And if he is unable to work again, he might discover something else to occupy his vocational need in some other way— perhaps a new hobby or interest that otherwise would not have been developed prior to the accident.

Although Fred's life has been dramatically altered by his physical injury and his former quality of life may be threatened, he may still find ways to enjoy his "new normal." With his inner resources and the support of others, he may have a good quality of life in spite of his disability. It is even conceivable that he may find a better quality of life than he had previously *because* of his disability.

Now consider the case of Wilma, a seventy-eight-year-old widow who has recently been diagnosed with AD. Although the disease can be seen primarily in terms of a threat to her intellectual well-being, it also has major implications for other dimensions of her well-being. Wilma lives alone and has four children; one daughter, Laurie, and several grandchildren live nearby. Wilma had been a meticulous housewife and bookkeeper. She took pride in managing her own affairs. Laurie prompted the medical evaluation that led to the diagnosis after noticing that Wilma's memory and organizational skills had been deteriorating over the past year. Laurie discovered that Wilma had forgotten to pay some bills and was not taking her medications routinely. She was no longer keeping up her home and cooking nutritious meals. Wilma had also withdrawn from her circle of friends and relatives and even stopped participating in her church choir. Laurie had long suspected her mother might have AD but had put off obtaining a medical evaluation until Wilma got seriously lost while driving her car one day. Wilma tearfully admitted that she was no longer able to trust her memory to make good decisions.

Unlike the sudden onset of Fred's physical disability, Wilma had been experiencing a gradual decline that had already diminished her well-being in significant ways. The diagnosis of AD confirmed that action was necessary to reverse the downward trend and to restore her to a better quality of life. Because of the very nature of her disease, she no longer had the capacity to do this on her own. Wilma's emotional well-being was threatened by AD as her identity as a competent, self-sufficient woman was under assault. She may react to her predicament with anger or she may feel relieved that she no longer has to struggle alone with her growing impairments. Other people will need to compensate for her and enable her to enjoy life now and in the future. For instance, someone else will need to ensure that she is taking her scheduled medications, eating properly, and paying her bills on time. Wilma might have to relocate to a place where her daily needs will be better met, but others will have to take the lead in this major decision. Wilma will need encouragement to participate in purposeful activities and social situations. Other people will have to make a conscious effort to continually boost her self-esteem. She will need frequent reminders that she is still a valued and lovable person despite her intellectual disability.

Laurie and other family members will have to assume increasing responsibility for Wilma's welfare, despite her protests. And yet, left to her own devices, Wilma's well-being would certainly continue to diminish. On the other hand, much can be done to improve her overall quality of life by addressing the problems that are already taking place. Wilma may eventually respond like another woman with AD who said, "I am not ready to die with this disease. I am living with it. There is still a whole lot of living to be done. I need the help of others to make my remaining time as meaningful as possible." Laurie and the rest of the family may look forward to seeing Wilma's life in a new and different way. Instead of looking on helplessly as Wilma struggles to cope with her symptoms, they may enable her to maximize her quality of life.

Dr. G. Allen Power is a geriatrician who is deeply disturbed by the negative stereotypes and stigma associated with AD. He thinks that the disease has become "medicalized" to the point of often ignoring the social and emotional needs of people with AD. In his book, *Dementia Beyond Drugs: Changing the Culture of Care,* he uses the language of physical disability to reframe how we think and behave toward people like Wilma.[2] The Americans with Disabilities Act legislated changes in physical design in our buildings and public spaces to accommodate the needs of disabled people. Ramps and elevators, for example, are now taken for granted to provide access to people in wheelchairs. Dr. Power argues that people with AD deserve "cognitive ramps" to ease their lives. Of course, he is not referring to physical modifications but rather to changes in the ways we relate to people with AD. How can we enable people with AD to use their remaining abilities and to minimize their disabilities? A wellness approach that puts each person's comfort and dignity at the center of all of our interactions is the key to a good life.

By adopting a positive outlook instead of the customary gloom-and-doom perspective about AD, it is possible to create opportunities for people with AD to enjoy a good quality of life. In other words, family, friends, and others involved with people who have AD can decide how they approach the disease and how they work toward positive solutions to its complex challenges. This is no easy task, for sure. And since the person with AD may live with this disease for many years ahead, providing the highest level of care is akin to running a marathon. It requires knowledge, patience, skill, compassion, and, above all, a team effort.

Relative Well-Being

The late Tom Kitwood, a psychologist who devoted himself to upholding the dignity of people with AD, was also highly critical of society's generally dim view of AD and the people living with the diagnosis. He viewed the traditional medical approach in mostly negative terms, as evidenced by the misuse of psychotropic drugs and other harmful ways of treating symptoms of the disease. Kitwood believed that the disease was potentially made worse by the dehumanizing attitudes toward people with AD that resulted in their diminished well-being. He knew that a person living with the disease would no longer enjoy the same quality of life that he or she had previously enjoyed. The gradual loss of intellectual skills made that impossible. Nevertheless, Kitwood thought that a person with AD still had the potential to enjoy life despite one's intellectual impairments and the resulting lifestyle changes. He strongly believed that everyone with AD was entitled to what he called "relative well-being."[3]

Kitwood was impressed by the capacity of people with AD to adapt to their symptoms. Moreover, their chances of adapting were greatly enhanced if they were surrounded by caring people who understood and supported their needs—especially their social and emotional needs. He called this "person-centered care"—high-quality interpersonal care that affirms personhood, resulting in the preservation of self. Conversely, Kitwood documented how people with AD were prone to a poor quality of life if their needs were not met, resulting in the loss of self. He saw people with AD being mistreated by others through demeaning words and actions. Poor care was chiefly responsible for their poor quality of life and the loss of self. Kitwood argued that the diminishment of personal identity often associated with AD was preventable by providing good care. He acknowledged that this requires a major shift in our usual ways of thinking about and relating to people with AD—viewing each person as a uniquely whole person in terms of all the dimensions of wellness.

A wellness approach to AD runs counter to the illness approach. Instead of focusing solely on one's needs and deficits, the primary goal is to maximize one's remaining capacities. The remainder of this book is about a positive approach aimed at enhancing personhood and quality of life. What might this look like in practical terms for someone with AD? Again, let's review each of the dimensions of wellness, keeping in mind that they are interconnected.

Emotional Wellness: The process of aging itself almost always involves losses and an assault on one's emotional well-being. Fears about becoming a burden to others run high. In addition to these losses, the symptoms of AD may further diminish one's sense of personal worth. The fear of becoming dependent may be fully realized. Feelings of insecurity, loneliness, sadness, depression, frustration, and anxiety are understandable. Deep questions may be raised: Am I a good person? Is life worth living? Is there hope?

To ensure emotional wellness among people with AD requires that other people believe that they can make a positive difference through their own words and actions. It also requires that every effort be made to minimize or prevent others from contributing to negative emotional well-being.

To ease the fears and worries of someone with AD, we must give him or her an abiding sense that at least one special person is readily available to serve as a confidante and best friend. This person is like a companion on the journey through the disease process. This "care companion" or "champion" can be counted on to ensure one's emotional comfort, strength, and security. This special person knows in detail the individual history of the person with AD, as well as his or her likes and dislikes, and communicates this important information to others. This companion educates and inspires other people to accept the role of preserving the emotional stability of the person with AD.

Any emotional problems are dealt with swiftly by looking at underlying causes and developing creative solutions. Returning to the case of Wilma, if she is distraught that she can no longer manage her own finances, there is no reason for daughter Laurie to completely take this responsibility from her. Wilma deserves opportunities to have a say in decisions affecting her. Although Laurie may do Wilma the favor of eliminating needless worry by managing all of her bills, for example, perhaps Wilma would prefer to write out a few checks monthly and review the bank statement with Laurie. In this way, Wilma may still feel good about keeping some control over her life and does not feel like a burden to her daughter.

Emotional wellness also means being free of major depression and anxiety. Individual counseling with a mental health professional such as a social worker or psychologist may be helpful in treating such problems. Drugs for these disorders should be prescribed cautiously due to side effects. Other types of psychotropic drugs used for treating mood and behavior should be used as a last resort due to their questionable benefits and side effects.

Intellectual Wellness: Because AD results in progressive loss of one's intellectual abilities, there is a tendency to think that not much can be done in this realm. It is useful to keep an open mind and explore a range of activities that may be worthwhile. The lack of solid evidence for using structured mental exercises and games has already been noted. However, these should not readily be dismissed unless the person with AD finds them to be too taxing or frustrating. The twin goals of any intellectual activity should be to promote use of one's remaining abilities and to enjoy performing those abilities instead of trying to improve memory.

It is important to choose intellectual activities that the person with AD finds pleasing, keeping in mind that the nature and intensity of these activities may change over time. For example, a person with AD may have once enjoyed reading books but can no longer remember story lines. However, much pleasure may be derived from reading short articles in newspapers and magazines or reading storybooks aloud to young children. Likewise, someone with AD may still enjoy playing cards and board games or enjoy the challenge of crossword or jigsaw puzzles. However, these activities may need to be simplified so that they are still enjoyable.

Everyday activities that require intellectual skills should also be encouraged such as performing household chores, preparing meals, and shopping. Simply engaging in a conversation is an intellectual activity—the normal give and take of conversation is not as easy as it appears! Because of memory and word-finding problems, someone with AD may not initiate a conversation but may communicate quite well under the right conditions (more on this topic in Chapter 8). Although AD inhibits the formation of new memories, memories of the distant past are usually well preserved in the early stages. Therefore, reminiscing may be a truly enjoyable intellectual activity. Scrapbooks, photo albums, home movies, recorded music, and other keepsakes will trigger conversations about one's personal background and historical events. Discussing the past may also offer valuable insights to younger people and help link the generations.

Intellectual activities that perhaps were not a focus of someone's past should be also explored to see if they strike a chord of enjoyment. Loads of small studies and anecdotal reports suggest the value of the creative arts for people with AD. Making art through painting or sculpting or simply enjoying art at museums can be highly satisfying activities that do not require short-term memory. Similarly, playing and listening to music can tap into old memories and lead to singing and dancing.

Social Wellness: Most of the intellectual activities noted above are social in nature. People with AD often withdraw from other people or customary activities. Whether this is a protective maneuver to shield them from feeling uncomfortable about their limitations or simply an effort to avoid situations that are taxing for the brain is not always clear. Regardless of the reason, loss of initiative to engage in social situations is fairly common, but being sedentary can breed a host of problems, including loneliness, apathy, sadness, boredom, and fear.

Other people often have to persuade the person with AD to engage in social activities. This may require skillful leadership and persistence in order to motivate someone to get outside their comfort zone (more on this topic in Chapter 6). Again, it is not advisable to push someone too hard. However, you should weigh the risks of social isolation versus the rewards of social engagement.

Consider again the case of Wilma who had withdrawn from her friends and family. Perhaps she had been feeling overwhelmed by the number of people and the confusion caused by the noise they create, and she felt she could no longer tolerate such situations. On the other hand, if someone made sure that Wilma was engaged in one-to-one conversations at social events instead of getting lost in a crowd of people, she might be more likely to enjoy herself.

A man with AD once told me that he had grown to dislike social situations until he and his wife devised a couple of clever strategies. First, she would take the lead in making introductions at any gathering in order to minimize his worry about remembering names. Second, he deliberately positioned himself in a corner of a room so that people could approach him only on an individual basis. This allowed him to converse easily without a chorus of voices taxing his brain. At the same time, his wife always kept a close eye to make sure that he was enjoying himself. If he got tired out, they had a pact to make a graceful exit. Pleasant gatherings increased his confidence and desire to stay socially engaged.

Physical Wellness: Most people with AD are older adults who are prone to have other chronic or acute illnesses or medical conditions. It is advisable to closely follow the recommendations of health-care providers to identify and manage these conditions and optimize one's physical well-being. In light of the growing link between heart health and brain health, every effort should be made to promote a good cardiovascular system. Adhering to a medication regime and a healthful diet are key elements of physical wellness (more on this topic in Chapter 7). Imagine the dire consequences for Wilma, for example, if she forgot to take vital medications or to eat regularly.

It is also important to take part in physical activities to increase endurance, strength, balance, and flexibility through regular exercise. Again, it is not known if exercise can help in slowing down the progression of AD. However, people with AD often develop difficulties with mobility that can result in falls, injuries, and death. Efforts to stay physically active may reduce the risk of mobility issues. Walking, jogging, and cycling are excellent forms of exercise and require minimal expense. A stationary bike, a treadmill, weights, or other equipment may be easy to use at home with proper supervision. Someone with AD can easily get some exercise simply by performing chores around the home such as vacuuming or doing yard work.

Structured exercise classes are available through community centers, health clubs, and recreational programs. These venues probably require someone to assist the person with AD to negotiate the surroundings and activities. For example, one woman with AD stuck to her routine of swimming three times weekly, thanks to her swimming partners at the local pool. A man with AD worked out regularly at a gym under the guidance of a personal trainer. Organized games that rely on motor skills such as bowling, shuffleboard, and croquet may also be therapeutic. And thanks to technology, someone with AD can engage in a variety of virtual sporting events at home like tennis, bowling, and golf. It is common today for retirement communities to engage their residents in such physical activities through the video game consoles known as the Wii and Xbox Kinect.

Like all the other dimensions of well-being, it is essential for the person with AD to choose those physical activities that he or she finds most enjoyable. In addition, having one or more people available to promote and guide these activities may be critical to successfully engaging someone in the achievement of optimal well-being.

Spiritual Wellness: This dimension concerns an appreciation for the wonders of the universe and connectedness to someone or something beyond oneself. For most people, organized religion provides a pathway to God and spiritual wellness, while others find nonreligious pathways such as nature, music, and art. For example, author Ed Voris speaks of his spiritual renewal after the onset of his AD in *Conversations with Ed*: "I can see and hear all the birds and animals that I didn't see or hear before. I don't think it's misleading to say that I'm unquestionably happier and fuller with less."[4]

For people with AD with faith traditions such as Christianity, Judaism, or Islam, a rich array of religious practices may be available to help them tap into long-term memories. Familiar prayers, readings, rituals, and hymns may be well preserved and recalled for personal and group worship. Catholics, for example, may well remember how to use rosary beads to repeat a series of prayers memorized decades ago. The predictable order of worship in churches, synagogues, and mosques may be comfortingly familiar. Participating in religious activities should be encouraged if they were once part of a person's heritage. People with AD who have lost touch with their religious roots may find spiritual solace in reconnecting to their faith tradition.

Vocational Wellness: This dimension refers to one's "calling" in life and sharing of personal talents. Too often people with AD lose confidence, feeling that they can no longer make contributions to others and the world. One's personal identity as a parent, grandparent, sibling, confidante, friend, helper, artist, singer, musician, or poet may be threatened as the disease takes its toll on intellectual skills. The major task of providing care to a person with AD is to help preserve that person's identity. Like other dimensions of well-being, the vocational dimension requires that we see personhood in social rather than in individual terms. Other people, especially the "care companion," need to provide opportunities for the person with AD to continue to make contributions of time and energy.

Recall again the case of Wilma who had stopped singing in her church choir. Perhaps this activity had been a primary way for her to contribute to her religious community. With the encouragement and practical help of others, however, Wilma could likely resume this activity. Not only would regaining her status as a choir member boost her self-esteem, but in doing so, she would also reap its spiritual benefits and restore her connections with members of her community.

Wholeness

Anyone seeking a medical solution to the problem of AD inevitably comes to the realization that there are no quick or easy answers. The biology of the disease is far more complex than Dr. Alzheimer could have imagined more than a century ago. Brain science is still a relatively young field. One neuroscientist used this analogy in regard to AD: "We are still at the foothills of our understanding and we have mountains yet to climb." Slow but steady scientific progress is being made. Of course, better funding for research is imperative to making further advances. In the meantime, there is much that can be done to enhance the quality of life for someone with AD through human ingenuity, skill, and compassion.

This chapter begins the shift in focus from a strictly medical approach to AD to a broader approach that encompasses all the dimensions of personal well-being. This broader approach allows for the person with AD to be seen as whole person who happens to have a disability due to a brain disease. This broader approach also allows for you and other people to play an active role in preserving this person's identity and well-being.

Someone with AD needs to be reminded by other people that he or she should not be defined by one's illness. Having a chronic illness, particularly late in life, is now commonplace. A person with AD is more than an intellect that is being compromised by a mysterious disease. Like anyone, a person with AD is multidimensional, with a rich personal background and a unique personality. And like anyone, a person with AD is greater than the sum of his or her parts—intellectual, physical, emotional, social, spiritual, and vocational. In some circles, this essential self is known as the soul. Despite a desire for perfection, we all have flaws or deficits, but they do not make us less than a whole person. It is this deep understanding about human nature that enables families, friends, and other care partners to provide a good life to someone with AD and to give meaning to this challenging experience. This positive perspective offers someone with AD true hope—not that the disease can be cured but confidence that others will offer security, kindness, and love when so many things are changing, both outside and within. The next section of this book addresses some of the practical details of this special type of care.

PART II

Giving Care

5 What Is It Like to Have Alzheimer's Disease?

What we see

depends upon where we sit.

• • • Ram Dass

Even though individuals with AD share many of the same symptoms, their unique personalities, backgrounds, and lifestyles greatly influence the ways in which they respond to their disease. Someone's past problem-solving style and coping strategies may well carry over to the present challenges resulting from AD. Then again, changes in one's memory and thinking may alter one's perceptions in ways that others find confounding. For example, someone with AD may not be bothered by the symptoms whereas his or her spouse may be deeply troubled by them. It is therefore crucial for you and others to first understand how the person with AD perceives his or her symptoms and how these symptoms affect his or her daily life. Understanding the individual's perspective can be very useful for you, the family members and friends, in the important work of adjusting your expectations to match the person's needs.

In this chapter, I focus on how people living with the disease experience it in different ways. To this end, I offer an assortment of personal stories to show how varied the experience of AD can be.

Unlike the growing body of literature by survivors of medical conditions such as cancer and stroke, relatively little material is available about the experience of living with AD. Because of the nature of the disease, people with AD have difficulty remembering and expressing their thoughts and feelings in customary ways. Their self-reflection is limited by forgetfulness. It should not be surprising, then, that although millions of people have experienced this disease, fewer than twenty people have written books about it. Those who do usually do so with the help of loved ones (see the Resources section at the back of the book for a list).

Fortunately, an increasing number of people in the early stages of AD are coming forward to share their personal experiences in public forums, newspaper articles, television and radio interviews, documentary films, educational videos, and of course, blogs and websites. For more than a decade, the publication *Perspectives: A Newsletter for Individuals with Alzheimer's or a Related Disorder* has given voice to people with the disease. (Contact lsnyder@ucsd.edu for this free quarterly newsletter.) People with Alzheimer's and other dementias as well as their supporters have also been linked through a Web-based organization, Dementia Advocacy and Support Network International (www.dasninternational.org). I suggest that anyone who cares for someone with AD would benefit from these first-person accounts.

Many novels and films have included stories about people with Alzheimer's disease, but none has been as popular as the best-selling book *Still Alice,* written from the perspective of a woman with AD.[1] Although a work of fiction, author Lisa Genova used her background in neuroscience and her family history with the disease to write a compelling story about Alice, a Harvard professor diagnosed with AD at age fifty. The novel chronicles the progression of Alice's early symptoms and the impact of her diagnosis on her career, family, marriage, and identity. The story about the unfolding of her disease and the ensuing personal drama offers great insight into the subjective experience of AD.

The fact that only a handful of people with AD have produced books suggests that they are exceptional individuals with a high degree of awareness about their disease (see the Resources section for a complete list of these books). While their insights may offer important clues about the experiences of others with the disease, it is a mistake to expect everyone with AD to have the high degree of insight that these individuals have shown. Still, all of these stories are worth reading since they may give you a better understanding of your loved one's experience and help you cope more effectively.

Some Common Experiences and Feelings

The published accounts by those with AD are uniquely personal but have some themes in common. These authors often describe feelings of alienation, loneliness, and fear; yet on a positive note, they also convey a deepened appreciation for life's simple pleasures. In *Partial View: An Alzheimer's Journey,* former history professor Cary Henderson describes his sense of alienation from others:

> Being dense is a very big part of Alzheimer's. Although I'm not as bad as I sometimes am, it comes and goes. It's a very come-and-go disease. When I make a real blunder, I tend to get defensive about it; I have a sense of shame for not knowing what I should have known. And for not being able to think things and see things that I saw several years ago when I was a normal person—but everybody by this time knows I'm not a normal person, and I'm quite aware of that.[2]

He also describes his sense of loneliness: "I think one of the worst things about Alzheimer's disease is that you are so alone with it. Nobody around you really knows what's going on. And half the time, or most of the time, we don't know what's going on ourselves."[3]

Loneliness and alienation are also described by Robert Davis, a pastor forced into retirement by AD, in his remarkable book, *My Journey into Alzheimer's Disease*:

> As soon as my diagnosis was announced, some people became very uncomfortable around me. I realize that the shock and pain are difficult to deal with at first. It was strange that in most cases I had to make the effort to seek out people who were avoiding me and look them in the eye and say, "I don't bite. I am still the same person, but I just can't do my work anymore. I know that one of

these days I will not be in here anymore, but for now, I am still home in here, and I need your friendship and acceptance."[4]

In his personal account, *Show Me the Way to Go Home*, Larry Rose writes of feeling cut off from the mainstream of life: "I can feel myself sliding down that slippery slope. I have a sadness and anxiety that I have never experienced before. It feels like I am the only person in the world with this disease." He also expressed his growing tendency to distance himself from others as a result of feeling different:

> I am becoming more and more withdrawn. It is much easier to stay in the safety of my home, where Stella treats me with love and respect, than to expose myself to people who don't understand, people who raise their eyebrows when I have trouble making the right change at the cash register, or when I'm unable to think of the right words when asked a question. Maybe it would be easier for them if I didn't look so healthy.[5]

In her memoir, Christine Boden describes how her memory and thinking problems led her to feeling disconnected: "We can't help the way we are—we know that there is something terribly wrong with us, and we seem to be losing touch with even who we are. We need all the help we can get."[6]

Although feelings of alienation and loneliness are often mentioned in these personal accounts, perhaps most troubling are the experiences of fear. Robert Davis writes, "Perhaps the first spiritual change I noticed was fear. I have never really known fear before. At night when it is total blackness, these absurd fears come.... The old emotions are gone as new uncontrolled, fearful emotions sweep in to replace them."[7] Cary Henderson notes that paranoia has crept into his psyche since the onset of AD: "I guess that the disease does make us kind of irrational. Sometimes it's out of fear, and sometimes it's being seemingly left out of things. But it's hard not to be suspicious, and I sure hope that nobody holds that against me."[8] In *Living in the Labyrinth*, Diana McGowin tells of a recurring fear that her husband might abandon her: "What would become of me? I needed his moral support and repeatedly sought his vow to take care of me for the rest of my life.

Upon receiving his assurance once again, I would inquire if he knew just how difficult keeping it may become in the future."[9]

Odd though it may seem, a deepened appreciation of simple pleasures is also a theme amidst these personal stories about feeling alienated, alone, and fearful. According to Robert Davis, "A journey into Alzheimer's is also a journey into the very basic simplicities of life."[10] In spite of a high degree of awareness of their symptoms and of the resulting changes in their lifestyles, a positive adaptation to the disease is evident. For example, Christine Boden notes:

> I am more stretched out somehow, more linear, more step-by-step in my thoughts... I'm like a slow-motion version of my old self— not physically but mentally. It's not all bad, as I have more inner space in this linear mode to listen, to see, to appreciate clouds, leaves, flowers.... I am less driven and less impatient.[11]

Larry Rose writes, too, about some benefits: "There have been many changes in my life since the onset of Alzheimer's, some of which I am not at all ungrateful for. I have more compassion for people, birds, deer, and the like. I have fallen more and more in love with Stella."[12] Diana McGowin also observes that her disease has given her a new perspective: "This knowledge enables me to savor life more openly and ravenously. I appreciate all good things more, whether they be trusted friends, cherished memories, nature's beauty, or physical pleasures."[13] The search for meaning and something positive in this personal experience of AD is repeated throughout Thaddeus Raushi's remarkably upbeat memoir, A View from Within. Although well aware of the changes and losses due to his disease, he chooses to adjust his attitude to fit the situation: "It has to do with little things in life elevated to a level of appreciation. It has to do with cherishing relationships."[14] The capacity for resilience in the face of hardship is striking throughout these personal accounts about living with AD.

Adaptation to AD may seem surprising given the daily frustrations imposed by the disease and its relentless nature. The awareness of decline in mental abilities is often coupled with appreciation of the remaining gifts in one's life. Those who find some peace in the midst of their confusion tend to challenge our assumptions about what it might feel like to live with the disease. Former President Ronald Reagan's letter to the American public in 1994 also illustrates this important point. He expresses concern about what the future may hold for his wife, yet the overall tone of his letter is not pessimistic. On the contrary, Mr. Reagan writes of his intention to continue enjoying outdoor activities and to stay in touch with friends and supporters. He ends his letter by noting, "I now begin the journey into the sunset of my life." This metaphor may jar our expectations about what he should be thinking or saying about having AD. Shouldn't he have felt angry or sad? Was he in a state of denial? Was he putting a political spin on a bad situation? How could he calmly face this disease, the same disease that caused his own mother's death?

Such questions are natural to ask. After all, memory and thinking skills are critically important—they help define who we are. Losing these skills may seem unimaginable. Many people believe that life would not be worth living with AD. It is important to distinguish our hypothetical reactions to AD from the real reactions of those living with the disease. Projecting our own negative feelings can create undue worry and increase the feelings of loneliness, alienation, and fear associated with the disease. Like many people with AD, I suspect Mr. Reagan was not hung up on comparing himself to the past nor was he worried about the future. He was content to live in the moment and had confidence that other people would attend to the details on his "journey into the sunset."[15]

To understand the state of mind of someone with AD, it is necessary to reexamine our expectations of how he or she should think or feel. To relieve the person with AD of the pressure to think or act "normally," we must accept the current reality of the individual—no matter how distorted it may seem. Trying to force people with AD into our version of reality does them a disservice and lowers their self-esteem by emphasizing their limitations instead of their remaining strengths. People with AD simply cannot keep pace with our old expectations, and under the circumstances we must adopt new ones that will accommodate the demands of the disease. Ethicist Stephen

Post stresses the need to reconsider our point of view in *The Moral Challenge of Alzheimer's Disease*:

> Because our culture so values rationality and productivity, observers easily characterize the life of persons with dementia in the bleakest terms.... The experience of the person with irreversible and progressive dementia is clearly tragic, but it need not be interpreted as half empty rather than as half full.[16]

Cary Henderson puts this sentiment in a uniquely personal way: "There are things that I wish I could do, but on the other side, there are still things that I can still do and I plan to hold on to them as long as I possibly can." Likewise, actor Charlton Heston eloquently conveyed his fighting spirit when he announced that he had been diagnosed with AD: "I'm neither giving up nor giving in.... I must reconcile courage and surrender in equal measure. Please feel no sympathy for me. I don't. I just may be a little less accessible to you, despite my wishes."[17]

Perhaps nobody else has defied stereotypes about living with AD more than Richard Taylor, forced to retire from his job as a psychology teacher when diagnosed at age fifty-eight. His symptoms have progressed in an unusually slow manner for more than a decade. He has turned his disease into a personal mission. He has become internationally known for his efforts to humanize the disease and advocate on behalf of others with the disease. His remarkable essays in *Alzheimer's from the Inside Out*, written with the aid of voice activated computer software, reveal a man bent on making sure that others treat him with respect and dignity. Rather than seeing his disease in tragic terms, he wants others to prevent the true tragedy: people like him being disabled and written off. He wants everyone with AD to have the benefit of a group of "best friends" who compensate for deficits and tap remaining abilities. He is fortunate to have found this caring community:

> My relationship with my spouse, my family, and my friends has broadened and in some ways deepened. We spend more time really being together. We talk more, we hug more, we cry more, we laugh more and harder and longer together.[18]

Varying Degrees of Awareness of Symptoms

At one time, it was assumed that everyone with AD was unaware of their memory loss and not troubled by it. Even today, some medical professionals mistakenly believe this to be true in all cases. Some people, such as those quoted above, are quite aware of their symptoms, while others seem oblivious of them. Still others with the disease fluctuate in their awareness, quite aware if they are taxed beyond their abilities but unaware if they are not challenged. For the most part, people with AD have a partial or limited insight into how the disease affects their lives. The disease often diminishes awareness about the nature and severity of symptoms, as if a dimmer switch has been lowered that reduces the ability to see things clearly.

No one is sure what accounts for these differing levels of awareness. Personality may play a role but does not alone account for such range of experiences. The extent and location of damage to the brain may also influence a person's degree of insight. Growing evidence, based on brain imaging studies, shows that the level of awareness is linked to the deterioration of the frontal lobe, the part of the brain associated with awareness, insight, and judgment. As AD advances over time, personal awareness of one's symptoms generally diminishes too—a strange sort of blessing.

How people with AD perceive their symptoms is key to understanding how they might receive your help. There is a good chance that someone who recognizes the limitations and effects of AD will see your help as necessary. Someone who is unaware of their symptoms may see your helpful efforts as unnecessary, demeaning, and intrusive. A trusting relationship with the person who has AD can enhance the level of cooperation, but trust alone will not win over someone who cannot see the need for help. Even though you have the best of intentions, you may not be able to persuade someone to accept your assistance.

For the minority of people with AD who are acutely aware of their disease, daily life can be quite frustrating, as the above-quoted authors illustrate. They may feel self-conscious and worry about making mistakes. Although they often try to compensate for or cover up their lapses, their efforts may fall short of their own expectations or those of others. They may become seriously depressed if they dwell on their failures, blame themselves for the problems caused by the disease, or say they feel stupid or make other self-deprecating remarks.

People with AD who are aware of their limitations may also take out their frustrations on loved ones. This is an understandable reaction but can be tough on those people. For example, in an article in the *Chicago Sun-Times,* a man with AD wrote about his displeasure with his wife's changing role in their marriage: "I get very angry with my wife. She's always bossing me around, telling me what I can do, what I can't do."[19] Likewise, a woman spoke of her misplaced anger about having the disease: "I'm not in charge. I'm not free to come and go as I've done in the past. I feel frequently that my husband thinks he owns me now. I guess part of my anger is being directed toward him when he is trying to fill in the gaps for me. I feel that I'm not my own person anymore."

In contrast, many people with AD express gratitude for the help of others. Noting his pride in his wife, one man confided to me:

> I'd like to get my memory better, but there's not much that can be done about it. I just do the best I can. My wife watches me like a hawk. Whatever has to be done, she'll say, "Joe, I'll do it" or "I'll help you do it." I get plenty of help. I know what she's doing. I've got the greatest wife in the world.

In a newsletter, a woman credits her husband's tact in helping her to cope: "He is my bulwark. The best thing about him is that he is willing to let me do as much as I can by myself. He does not hover over me and tell me I can't do things. Instead, he offers support and encouragement. I never feel inadequate when he's around."

Clearly, those who are aware of their disease vary in their response to living with its effects. Some are conflicted about asking for or receiving help. One woman with AD interviewed for the *Perspectives* newsletter (mentioned above) expresses mixed feelings: "I fought like hell—every single step—in getting help. I'd think, 'I don't need it yet,' or 'I don't want it now.' Then eventually I'd think, 'I really do need help now. It won't hurt me.' I'm always glad when I do get help. It's a slow process, I guess." This struggle between independence and dependence will be discussed again in the next chapter.

At the other end of the spectrum are those people who appear oblivious to their disease. Sometimes they are described as being in a state of denial, a common defense mechanism that shields the human psyche from painful realities. However, this description is generally not useful in understanding people with the disease. Faulty memory and judgment, not denial, lead many people with AD to believe that they are intact. They may not realize that they are forgetting names or places, or they may not be troubled by it. To put it simply, they forget that they forget. As a result, their frustration may be mild or even nonexistent. They firmly believe that all is well. For example, a man made this observation in describing the trouble he had performing his job: "I was not aware that I was having difficulties, but my difficulties were made plain when my supervisor pointed out my lapses in a very abrasive manner.... You cannot experience what you have forgotten." The following excerpts from interviews I conducted with people with AD further illustrate this lack of awareness.

An eighty-year-old retired railroad worker reports: "I'm slower than I was because I'm older. My wife says my memory is real bad, but I don't notice it." He goes on to explain, "I can do anything I always did. Maybe not as fast, but I do it. I still drive a car! My wife says I forget where I'm going, but I don't think so. She gets mad at me because I forget. She says that I don't do anything. She says I should be more active. It bothers her more than it bothers me."

A seventy-year-old homemaker explains, "I don't believe I have a memory problem because I have a better memory than the average person. I mean this sincerely. In fact, I have a better memory than my husband." About the impact of AD on her life she notes: "I do the same things I did all the time. I wash, I cook, I iron, and I shop. I try to manage as much as I can. I can forget things, but you know, I'm not a youngster anymore."

Confronting people who are oblivious about their impairments is not only pointless, but also may cause upset for all concerned. There is evidence that damage to the frontal lobe of the brain, chiefly responsible for judgment and awareness, may be responsible for this lack of awareness. It is best to blame this state of mind on the disease, rather than on the person. This situation is often puzzling, sometimes maddening, to family members, friends, and others who are eager to help those in need with practical issues such as finances. It is very difficult to elicit the cooperation of those who do not see the need for help.

In general, people who are either highly aware of their disease or completely oblivious to it are a minority of those with AD. For most people in the early stages, personal awareness fluctuates but generally remains at a lower level than expected. The disease appears to blunt personal insight about the nature and degree of cognitive decline. Most people don't dwell on their impairments, or they find ways to excuse them. And, yes, denial may play a role, too, as one man told me:

> Remarkably, a number of us with Alzheimer's are chipper. I'm not sure why. My guess is that having gotten the heavy news, we decide we will make the most of being with friends and family and of doing things we love to do. It's a prescription that people without Alzheimer's might try. I do not mean to suggest that people with Alzheimer's do not take the measure of our prospects…[but] a degree of denial is essential. Like somebody drinking hot coffee, we sip the truth of our condition carefully and gently.

The following interview excerpts illustrate the partial or low level of awareness that is fairly common among those in the early stages of the disease:

A seventy-five-year-old retired electrician reports:

> I've got memory problems. I'm not so sharp the way I used to be. I guess old age is creeping in, so we've got to take it whether we like it or not. A lot of people are worse off than I am, so I have to take it one day at a time and hope for the best."

He later says:

> I still don't see much difference in my life, you know. I worked as an electrician in a shop, so I always used my hands. I was pretty good, too. I'm still busy all the time. I got my home and my garden,

and I'm always fiddling around. I always find a job to do. I do what I'm familiar with, and if I'm asked to do something different, I can ask for advice.

A seventy-three-year-old retired teacher comments:

I've read about this disease. I don't have as much use for my memory as I used to. You see, the things I forget are the things I don't come in contact with anymore, I would say. If I forget, I either look it up or ask my husband, because we're both at home. I'll say, "Honey, I forgot this and that. Can you remember?" And he will help me remember.

Regarding her expectations for the future, she notes: "Well, I just hope that my health lasts the way it has. I hope I can live the way I am now in spirit and body, because I have a very good life."

Because of their inability to recall the recent past or plan ahead for the future, people with AD naturally tend to focus on the present and the distant past. Although cognizant of losses or changes, they often begin a gradual process of adaptation to their disease. Over time, people with AD generally seem to lower their expectations of their own abilities, instead of struggling to maintain former standards of thinking and doing things. As one woman noted about her mother with AD: "She knows that she doesn't remember and knows that she can't do certain things on her own. She takes it very calmly. It doesn't frustrate her the way it would frustrate me." As the recent past and future dwindle in importance, and other people assume responsibility for remembering and planning for them, affected people can experience the "here and now" more freely. The experience of living in the present moment takes on a deeper meaning. A woman with AD recounted an incident that enabled her to appreciate the present moment. After describing her mourning over "the loss of what was and what might be," she said:

One day as I fumbled around the kitchen to make a pot of coffee, something caught my eye through the window. It had snowed, and I had forgotten what a beautiful sight a soft, gentle snowfall could be. I eagerly dressed and went outside to join my son who was shoveling our driveway. As I bent down to gather a mass of those radiantly white flakes on my shovel, it seemed as though I could do nothing but marvel at their beauty. Needless to say, my son did not share in my enthusiasm. To him it was nothing more than a job; but to me it was an experience. Later, I realized that for a short period of time, God granted me the ability to see snowfall through the same innocent eyes of the child I once was, so many years ago. Jan is still there, I thought, and there will be wonders to behold in each new day. They will just be different now.

Clearly, how people with AD perceive their symptoms is highly individualized and may be radically different from our perception of what it might feel like to us. Furthermore, in trying to understand the thinking and behavior of people with AD, we can no longer rely on our past expectations or experiences with them. In fact, our past relationship with an individual may actually limit our insight into how the affected person is being challenged by the disease right now. This suggests that our prior assumptions about the relationship may no longer apply in light of current circumstances. A whole new way of thinking and acting is usually required to accommodate the changing world of someone with AD.

The Importance of Social Environment

Anyone who has ever become disabled, regardless of the underlying condition, experiences a sense of losing her or his place in the world. For people with AD this is true in both literal and figurative terms, since becoming disoriented about time and place is a common symptom. On another level, one's sense of self may feel threatened as connections to other people, places, and things start to slip over time. What was once familiar and routine can easily become unfamiliar and confusing. Therefore, it is vital for people with AD to have caring people who can help connect them to their environment. In fact, the presence or absence of caring people may be the most significant factor in determining the quality of life for someone with AD.

This feeling of becoming unmoored or disoriented was described in Dr. Alzheimer's original case report of Auguste Deter, the middle-aged woman with AD. This unfortunate woman was uprooted from her family and home in 1901 and placed in a psychiatric hospital in Frankfurt, Germany, until her death in 1905. According to Dr. Alzheimer's written notes, she often remarked, "I have lost myself." [20] Although her disease had caused her disorientation, the stark surroundings in which she lived most likely intensified it. There was little or nothing to give her a sense of normalcy or help her feel connected to her past life. No meaningful activities were offered to rekindle her interest or enjoyment in everyday life. In the impoverished lifestyle of a hospital, cut off from familiar people and activities, it was no wonder that Deter experienced a loss of self.

Although it has been more than a century since Dr. Alzheimer and Auguste Deter met, the importance of helping those with AD feel connected to the world and other people is still not completely understood. At one time it was believed that an individual's life before the onset of the disease had little or no bearing on his or her experience of AD. Moreover, it was believed that nothing could influence the progressive course of the disease and that quality of life would be marginal at best. In recent years, these assumptions have been challenged by the growing realization that much can be done to enhance the well-being of people with AD.

Some researchers have suggested that when family and friends compensate for the disabilities of the person with AD and promote remaining abilities, the rate of decline may be slowed. Just as an impoverished environment can intensify people's symptoms and diminish their quality of life, an enriched environment may positively influence their disease process and improve their quality of life. This requires great sensitivity about all the dimensions of their well-being and taking responsibility for meeting their needs. Rather than relying exclusively on medical treatments to improve the well-being of those with AD, we can instead focus on our personal interactions with them, which can often do far more to influence their quality of life. A good relationship is better than the most powerful drug.

What Do People with AD Really Need?

Although every person with AD is unique, and individual preferences must be respected, people with the disease generally share the same basic needs. In addition to the physical need for food, clothing, and shelter, people with AD require three other things to be relatively happy: intimacy, community, and meaningful activity.

Intimacy refers to closeness to and familiarity with other people, places, and things. In an intimate relationship such as a marriage or friendship, individuals care about one another and look out for one another's welfare. Intimacy is essential for emotional well-being. Without intimacy, fear and loneliness prevail. When the need for intimacy is not met, a host of real and imagined fears commonly take root in people with AD. They may fear losing control of their life or being abandoned by family and friends. One man noted that his wife with AD became obsessed with locking the doors to their home because she was worried about intruders. A woman with AD told me one day, "I worry that my husband is having an affair and will leave me." They may fear becoming dependent and becoming a burden to others. A man with AD worried about being a burden to his daughter: "The thing I hate the most is always asking her for reminders. She's got better things to do than looking after me. She's got a life of her own, after all." Whether or not these worries are warranted, they are quite real to the person with AD. Intimacy through physical touch, as well as staying in touch with others, helps someone with AD to overcome these fears.

Sometimes this need for intimacy is exaggerated, as seen in those who cling to or "shadow" their loved ones. Just being in the physical presence of a trusted person at all times may offer reassurance to someone with AD who otherwise feels fearful while alone or with strangers. Likewise, feeling connected to a familiar and safe place such as one's home can also be comforting. Again, this may be exaggerated in the form of the person with AD resisting invitations to go outside the home. Even closeness with pets or other favorite things can offer comfort. Cary Henderson's personal account includes much praise for his dog as well as a suggestion for others with AD: "I sort of think that anybody with Alzheimer's could benefit by a friendly little dog.

Somebody they can play with and talk to—it's kinda nice to talk to a dog that you know is not going to talk back. And you cannot make a mistake that way." Larry Rose's story of living with AD is also filled with funny and touching references to his constant companion, a pot-bellied pig named Floyd.

People with AD need intimacy perhaps more than ever. As they gradually lose their customary ways of connecting with other people and the world, they need others to reach out to them and help them feel connected. And because their sense of initiative often wanes, others must extend themselves to meet this need for intimacy in active ways. Intimate relationships make people with AD feel safe and allow them to enjoy being known and appreciated.

Community refers to a sense of belonging to a group with whom one shares a common bond. This community can consist of just one other person, a family, or a larger group of people who can see beyond superficial realities to the value of each person. Community is essential for emotional well-being. People with AD may feel cut off from their family, friends, and neighbors due to their forgetfulness and other impairments. Like the lepers of biblical times, they often feel rejected, unwelcome, or out of place in a society that places a high value on self-reliance, productivity, and intellectual prowess. People with AD often think and act differently from those who are considered "normal." They may feel alienated and embarrassed when they fail to remember names or cannot complete a simple task. A man with AD admitted to me: "I used to be full of self-confidence, but now I'm quite conscious of making mistakes. I do not want to appear foolish in front of other people." A true community, however, recognizes the diversity of human experiences and allows everyone to be treated in humane and dignified ways—especially those who have a disability.

People with AD need reassurance that they are accepted for who they are and not for what they can do. Belonging to a caring community means that someone with AD is accepted without the usual conditions being met. Their limitations are downplayed, while their remaining strengths are celebrated. The personal worth of someone with AD can be sustained if others share this vision of a caring and inclusive community. Family members and friends can learn to create this warm and friendly atmosphere, and thereby enrich the lives of everyone involved. The need for community is often met in support groups for people with AD by virtue of their shared concerns. One woman praised her support group for people in the early stages of AD, saying: "I am at peace when I'm with my group. I can be myself without pretending that I am 100 percent. The group has been my lifeline. Everyone there understands what it feels like to be lost and forgetful. It makes no difference to us."

Finally, people with AD need to be involved in *meaningful activities,* an essential aspect of vocational well-being. Without meaningful activities, people with AD are at risk for loneliness, boredom, and helplessness. Preconceived notions about productive work or hobbies must be replaced with new ideas for activities that suit their abilities and disabilities. If placed in a situation where they can do little or nothing for themselves, they will feel inadequate and slip into passivity. But if given opportunities for active participation, no matter how small their role may be, affirmation and success are possible. Self-esteem can be restored and maintained.

Activities are the everyday stuff of life. Cooking a meal, making a bed, cleaning a room, singing a tune, shopping for food, caring for a pet, and taking a walk are the kind of informal activities that can give life meaning for the person with AD. Such ordinary things can highlight a person's remaining abilities and create opportunities to give to others instead of always being the recipient of care. People with AD can do some of these activities alone, but more often they need the encouragement and support of other people. Consequently, intimacy and community are reinforced through engaging in meaningful activities together. Christine Boden summed up this need for connectedness in her personal account of living with AD: "I want to carry on drinking in the beauty of this world and feel the love of my family and friends. Even if I might not remember these experiences very long, I still want to have them. Surely, remembering an experience doesn't constitute the sole enjoyment of that moment!"[21]

People with AD depend on other people to see the world through their eyes and ensure that their needs for intimacy, community, and meaningful activity are met. They need at least one caring person to step forward to ensure that these needs are met. One or more people must assume responsibility for being a special companion, care partner, best friend, or leader. The fact that you are reading this book suggests that you may be the primary person in this important role. In the next chapter, I will address how you can best serve your loved one with AD in your role as a leader.

What Some Family Members Have to Say

The following quotes from relatives of people with AD illustrate how caring and compassionate relationships are at the heart of meeting needs. More advice from relatives of people with AD will be shared in Chapter 13.

Geri comments about her mother with AD:

> She needs for us to say, "It's okay to be like this, Mom. We still like you. People still want to be with you." We have to give her a push to get back into society, or she would stay home all of the time. We make sure that she eats and her clothes are clean. We try to make sure she does things for herself too.

Marge makes this observation about her husband with AD: "He needs me to be in charge. If that appears difficult for me, he feels guilty that he is a burden to me. He needs to know that I'm okay with this and that I'm in it for the long haul."

George offers this assessment of his wife: "More than anything else, she needs to be kept happy. I don't want her to be in any situation where she is befuddled. I look out for her and for myself as well."

Fred simply notes about his wife: "She needs for me to keep cool. If I get upset, so does she."

Mary says this about her husband:

> He needs my love and affection. He needs direction, too. He will do anything I ask of him, but he will not volunteer to do anything. I told him today to go to the local gas station to get the gas can filled for the lawnmower and to pick up a newspaper, too. He got

the newspaper but forgot about the gas can. I should have known better.

Frank says this about his sister: "It isn't the practical help so much as the moral support. I would never think of harping on her because she cannot remember a name. If she wants to tell a story but can't remember the names of the people involved, I tell her to go ahead anyway."

Phillip notes: "My mother always wants to be busy. She lives alone, and if she is by herself for more than a day, she is not happy. She needs my time and support."

Sally describes her approach with her husband:

> He needs gentle reminders. I try to make light of it. I know he needs lots of love and praise from me. I leave him alone unless I know he's really struggling with something. If I jump in too fast, he gets aggravated. I would rather have him succeed on his own and feel good about his accomplishments.

. . . .

These family members did not come to a sudden understanding of their unique position in the life of a loved one with AD. Rather, with time and experience, they gradually adjusted to their new role. This process required a profound shift in how they viewed their relationship with the individual, who was changing due to the disease. They slowly learned how to make changes to fit the situation. In the next chapter, I will address many of the important aspects of these changing roles and responsibilities.

6 How Relationships, Roles, and Responsibilities Change

*My mother and I have gotten closer
because of this diagnosis.*

Tyler Summitt, son of legendary women's
basketball coach Pat Summitt

Since the dawn of human time, people have understood the need to be connected to others for the sake of protection, companionship, and enjoyment. We are born into relationships and choose them throughout our lifetime. Relationships are in our DNA. The notion of the rugged individual who stands alone is a modern myth that belies the reality that all of us are connected at some level. The personal and social are intertwined. AD puts this reality to the test. Although an individual has the disease, other people will be affected—some will choose to be involved in providing care and some will opt out. Regardless of how others respond, the diagnosed person needs help to cope with the disabling effects of the disease that threaten his or her well-being.

AD inevitably leads to changes in relationships. Similar to the progression of the disease, these changes are subtle at first but slowly become profound. People with AD can no longer function as they once did. Their communication and reasoning skills gradually falter. They can no longer handle responsibilities that they once took for granted. As a result, you must learn to accept their declining abilities and make adjustments. Your relationship with the affected person cannot continue as it once was. You will have to change your expectations of what she or he can and cannot do independently, compensate for the disabilities, and assume a growing number of responsibilities. As one woman said about her husband with AD, "We are the ones who must change. He cannot and will not change to suit us." This requires a major shift in attitudes and behaviors.

In this chapter, I discuss your unique role in the life of the person with AD as well as the changing nature of your relationship with relatives, friends, and others. If your spouse or partner has AD, the sad truth is that your relationship will never be the same again. You will need to assume a more-active role in your relationship than ever before. If your mother or father has AD, your relationship with your parent will also change. The time and energy that you will need to devote to various things formerly done by your parent will increase over time. And your involvement with a spouse or parent who has AD will probably affect all your other relationships as well—with other relatives, with friends, and with coworkers. This disease is like a pebble cast into a pond with ripples being felt by lots of people, especially those nearby.

Accepting the Diagnosis

The first step is to accept that the diagnosis of AD is a permanent reality. It is natural in the beginning to want to deny this—denial is the human psyche's way of protecting us from feeling the terrible effects of painful situations. It allows time for the news to sink in. You may initially overlook or excuse the symptoms of AD until something forces the issue of getting a diagnosis. You may then doubt the diagnosis, and seek a second or third opinion. Such reactions are understandable and normal. Doubt and denial initially enable you to prepare emotionally for the reality and the practical implications of living with the disease. Keep this in mind as you deal with others who may have difficulty accepting the news or who downplay the seriousness of the situation.

Denial is often reinforced by the misleading—or seemingly absent—symptoms of the disease. After all, the person with AD may appear physically healthy. One man commented about his wife, "Because she looks as good as she does, it's really hard to believe that her brain is really sick." A daughter noted, "It's easy to overlook my mother's need for help. She looks just fine, in spite of her difficulties. In fact, she looks much better than the average person her age. It's tempting to forget that she really has Alzheimer's."

The fluctuating nature of the symptoms can also make you wonder about the diagnosis. There may be days when the person with AD is like his or her old self much of the time. So many abilities may be intact that you may be led to minimize the person's impairments. Gloria Hoffman addressed this point in the educational video, *Caring About Howard:* "There was a time that I was on such a roller coaster. He'd be real good one day, and I'd think, 'Is there anything wrong with him?' And then the next day, he couldn't remember anything. One day I'd be elated and then the next day I'd be down." [1] The analogy of a roller coaster ride is often used to describe the experience of living with someone with AD. The ups and downs defy our usual expectations for consistent behavior. One husband confided to me:

> Even though she was diagnosed with Alzheimer's a year ago, I keep having this internal argument about whether she has this disease. Upon the recommendation of a therapist, I have started telling myself once a day, "Yes, she does have Alzheimer's disease." Saying this seems to be helping to quiet my mind.

Your reluctance to accept the diagnosis may be reinforced by the person with AD, who could be adamant about holding on to personal freedom and autonomy. Values of self-reliance and individualism are deeply rooted in our culture. We seldom, if ever, wish to appear dependent on others for anything. Men in particular have traditionally associated dependence with personal weakness and a threat to their masculinity. And women, who have traditionally been responsible for caring for others, may resist being cared for themselves. One woman with AD explained this dilemma by saying, "When you have always been a person who likes to give assistance, it's hard to be on the receiving end."

Because of the negative connotations of dependence, it is understandable that people with AD may be reticent to ask for help or may resist helpful overtures. Some people with AD express this desire for independence in the form of resentment or hostility toward those who are offering help. At times, there may be an apparent contradiction between their desire for independence and their need to be helped with certain things. The person with AD may give mixed signals: wanting help, wanting to be independent, wanting to be accommodated, or wanting to be treated normally. This is a dilemma for those who give care and those who receive care. One man with the disease articulated this inner struggle when he told me, "The strange thing about living with this disease is that you've got to fight it and accept it at the same time." When famed women's basketball coach Pat Summitt was diagnosed with AD, she bristled at the thought of dependence on others. However, she reluctantly accepted the changes in her life as described in her autobiography *Sum It Up:* "The only way to deal with trouble of this magnitude was to face it—and to admit that I would need a lot of help.... But in facing weakness, you learn how much there is in you, and you find real strength."[2]

As a partner in care, you should not expect to take in the fullness of the implications of the disease immediately. Understanding—and acceptance—usually occurs in fits and starts. You may feel that you have little or no time in your life for the demands of the disease. Other priorities may take precedence over or compete with the needs of the person with AD. However, you and the affected person will be better off in the long run if you begin now to assume a leadership role in your relationship. The person with AD may suffer adverse consequences if you do not take into account how the disease is disrupting his or her life. By accepting the diagnosis and its life-changing effects, your ability to control your reactions to disease-related changes will improve significantly. The person with the disease will also benefit from your enlightened perspective. You will begin, in a sense, to make room for the disease without letting it completely dominate your life. Try not to feel overwhelmed by the current challenges or those that lie ahead. Time allows for plenty of on-the-job training in learning how to care for someone with AD.

Stepping into the Leadership Role

Since the person with AD no longer possesses the mental skills to be completely independent, a special brand of leadership is called for. At least one person must assume overall authority for ensuring the well-being of the person with AD, but it is best to include others, too, if at all possible. Much work is involved in addressing basic physical needs like food and shelter as well as meeting needs related to other dimensions of personal well-being that have been described. You need not be afraid of taking on this important leadership role or a major part of it, although it may feel awkward at first. The person with AD needs your help. Someone has to assume this responsibility or else trouble will ensue. If possible, it is best to share this critical role or delegate responsibilities to others who are willing to help and support your efforts.

Whether the person with AD is your spouse, parent, sibling, or in-law, a shift in the balance of power must occur in your relationship. You may feel uncomfortable at first with the term "power." Yet the dynamics of power, influence, and authority exist in every relationship. They can be used constructively or destructively, for good or ill. The change in power balance derives from the fact that the person with AD needs protection from the risks posed by the disease and can no longer meet her or his needs alone. Because of impairment in memory, thinking, or other brain functions, the person with AD no longer has intellectual equality with others. Coming to terms with this unfortunate reality is a difficult step in the right direction. As one person's role in the relationship changes and personal control diminishes, the other person's role must change in corresponding ways.

Any person giving direction and assuming greater responsibility in a relationship is exercising more power than the other person. This does not mean, however, that the dignity of the person with AD should be diminished or ignored. On the contrary, preserving his or her dignity becomes the utmost priority. In taking leadership, your job is not to dominate the life of the person with AD, but to help minimize the affected person's disabilities and maximize his or her remaining abilities. This implies not only caring *for* the person with AD but also caring *about* the person. Ultimately, the leadership role is about meeting the needs of the other person in dignified and respectful ways. That's why the term *care partner* seems more fitting than *caregiver*.

It takes self-confidence to assume leadership on behalf of another adult. It also takes extraordinary empathy, patience, and understanding to exercise this powerful role in a loving way. Despite the inequality of the partnership, the self-esteem of the person with AD must be upheld. Otherwise, feelings of embarrassment, depression, and frustration may arise, and conflicts may develop. In *Counting on Kindness: The Dilemmas of Dependency,* Wendy Lustbader describes the finesse required of the leader:

> The best assistance is that which is unobtrusive. Helpers who quietly get things done, rather than announcing their efforts, leave a dependent person's pride intact. The indebtedness position is not emphasized, and no mention is made of special accommodations. The fact of helplessness then recedes into the background, where it can reside without harming the person's self-esteem.[3]

Sensitivity to the feelings of the person being helped can lead to mutual understanding and cooperation. A caring leader seeks first to find out, "What can you do or what would you like to be helped to do?" instead of "What do you want or what can I do to help you?"

Knowing how and when to help out completely, partially, or not at all also requires you to think on your feet. Sometimes it may seem more efficient for you to take over a task completely. At the same time, by doing so, you may be ignoring the remaining abilities of someone with AD. You may reason, "I can fix a meal in half the time it takes him so I might as well do it by myself," even though the person with AD may derive satisfaction from playing a part in meal preparation. At the other extreme, you may assume that a certain task can be done independently, causing the person with AD to struggle needlessly. You may think, "She can still manage paying those bills by herself" when, in fact, she may silently wish for relief from this stressful work. Understanding the different levels of dependence and independence requires much insight into the needs and preferences of the affected person. At the same time, you cannot overlook the limits on your own time, energy, and patience. Balancing all these practical and personal needs can be a real juggling act.

A good metaphor for the changing relationship between you and the person with AD is the relationship between two ballroom dancers. When a couple dances, the roles of leader and follower are carefully orchestrated. A good leader dances in a way that enables the follower to be led almost effortlessly. The leader's cues may be so subtle that the follower may not appear to be led at all. The couple dances together gracefully as each partner cooperates in playing his or her part. In your relationship with a person with AD, you may be called on to change roles from follower to leader.

Another thing about your relationship is that you can no longer take for granted that the person with AD will remember the proper steps. You must now take a more active role in the dance. You must learn when to step in and when to step back. Fluctuations in symptoms will often make it hard for you to gauge when to step in to offer help and when to step back and refrain from helping. A woman described this problem in relation to her husband with AD: "Perhaps hardest is the contradiction between his need for independence and his need for help with some things. This leads him to accuse me, on the one hand, of treating him like a child and, on the other, of not being sensitive to his needs."

It may take a long time—months or even years—for you to learn a new set of "mental gymnastics," even though you may know that a different way of relating is now required. It is difficult to make this change. For example, a daughter whose mother was diagnosed with AD five years ago told me about her tendency to still correct her mother if she says something off kilter when it's pointless to do so. The daughter joked, "Sometimes I forget that she has this memory problem!"

The transition to your new leadership role can evolve over time. In its early stages, the disease does not require that you assume a full-time position as a provider of care. On a practical and emotional level, it is important to keep in mind the limits of your leadership role at this stage. One man shared his thoughts with me about his limited but central role during the early stage of his wife's disease:

> I purposely don't think of myself as a "caregiver," as the word implies a total dependence on her part. This may be a matter of semantics, but I try to differentiate between what she needs for me to do for her and what she can do for herself. So far, the latter far

outweighs the former. When that switch takes place, I guess I will have become a caregiver.

Fortunately, since AD progresses very slowly, in most cases you can make the shift in your role as leader bit by bit. The sooner the shift in roles takes place, however, the better it will be for the person with AD. If you are assertive without being domineering, helpful without being overbearing, and kind without being patronizing, then the person with the disease is likely to respond positively to your good intentions.

When Your Partner Has AD

If your spouse or partner has AD, how will your new role as leader affect your relationship? The answer to this question may well depend on how you worked out the terms of your relationship in the past. On the one hand, if you tended to be more the leader in the past, then you may possess the experience and self-confidence to assume the responsibilities that your loved one with AD once managed. On the other hand, if the person with AD was more the leader in your relationship, then you are more likely to have difficulty adjusting to the leadership role. A man with AD described the changing roles in his marriage: "There are times when I have a difficult time doing things, and I ask for her help. I guess that's different from what it used to be. Years ago, I was the macho man. I was the guy who did everything. Now she does most things, and I don't like that. But it's something that has to be done." He later noted, "Most of the time she's right, but sometimes I just want to do what I want to do." If you and your partner were more or less equals in the past, then you may be equipped to accept the changes occurring now. You can draw upon the strengths of your past relationship to move forward.

Likewise, if you have enjoyed a long and happy relationship, your history together may empower you to deal with present and future challenges. However, even the longest unions, lasting fifty or sixty years, are tested by AD. If you had a turbulent marriage, for example, then you may dread caring for a spouse with the disease. On the other hand, if you remarried late in life and didn't have many years together before your spouse got the disease, then you may wonder if you have the commitment to continue in the relationship. In addition, your spouse's children by a former marriage may not readily accept your leadership role. Anything less than a strong relationship may be threatened by the demands imposed by the disease. Mixed feelings are bound to arise. There is great potential for emotional upset and relationships may become strained. Getting the help you need to navigate such difficulties is paramount.

In committed relationships there is an expectation that each person will do his or her part to nurture the other person. Mutuality and reciprocity are inherent aspects of the marriage agreement or long-term partnership. Unfortunately, AD no longer allows the spouse or long-term partner with the disease to fulfill his or her part of the nurturing bargain. This is often a sad and painful reality for the well spouse, whose partner can no longer participate fully in the marriage or make decisions in traditional ways. While new ways of communicating, solving problems, and expressing love can be discovered, the burden of breaking old habits and creating new ones falls on the shoulders of the well partner.

Someone with AD who was your friend, helper, advisor, and intimate companion may no longer be capable of continuing in these roles. And you will no longer be able to take for granted the practical tasks formerly carried out by your partner. You will now need to assume those responsibilities or delegate them to someone else. Here are some examples of this dynamic:

- A husband noticed that his wife could no longer prepare hot meals safely and needed supervision: "I had never cooked a meal in our fifty-two years of marriage. Now I'm the chief cook."

- A wife realized that her husband could no longer manage their finances: "He resented my help at first. I did not have the skills or experience to deal with brokers, but I eventually caught on. I did not even know how to balance a checkbook until I learned that he was making a mess of things."

- A husband said, "It may sound funny, but I did not know how to operate the washing machine. When my wife could no longer do this job, I had to ask my daughter how to do the laundry."
- A wife said, "He did all of the grocery shopping after he retired. Then he began to forget items at the store, so I had to resume this responsibility."
- After a wife observed her husband's erratic driving, she said, "He had always been the main driver until I realized that he was endangering himself and others. Now I have taken over as the full-time driver, in spite of his resistance."

New or increased responsibilities for such practical tasks are a major part of the changes in the marital relationship. However, expressions of intimacy, including sex, are likely to change, too. Intimacy rests on many interconnected abilities that are impaired by AD. These include the capacity to convey one's thoughts and feelings and to comprehend verbal and nonverbal communication. The overall quality of the relationship suffers when the partner with AD can no longer give or receive intimacy in his or her usual way. Furthermore, for reasons not fully understood, sexual interest and function often wane among people with AD. Sexual desire in the healthy partner may also diminish because of the many changes taking place in the relationship.

Couples who continue to find satisfaction in their relationship, sexual and otherwise, usually do so by redefining the terms of their commitment. Instead of expecting a fifty-fifty partnership, the well partner typically accepts the other partner's limitations and creates new opportunities for shared meaning and closeness. Healthy relationships grow from the flexibility of both partners in responding to changing circumstances in the course of their life together. Although the person with AD may no longer have the capacity to make adjustments, the other partner can, in effect, take the lead in renegotiating their commitment, so that both feel comfortable with their changing roles and responsibilities. Again, a good lead dancer knows how to do this with finesse, but it stems from a lot of practice.

Many committed people who are not married are affected in similar ways when one partner develops AD. For a variety of reasons, a growing number of older people choose to live together without getting married. They may meet late in life after the death of a spouse or a divorce and may decide to live together, but may not wish to formalize their commitment in a marriage. Such partners may have a moral obligation to each other, but they often lack the legal and financial protections afforded to married couples. Likewise, older gay and lesbian couples may have a long-term relationship but without the same rights as married couples. Furthermore, most same-sex couples have paid a high emotional price for their sexual orientation. Their extended families may be split over their lifestyle and over accepting their lifelong partner. However, partners in such relationships confront issues similar to those faced by married couples when one partner has AD. The changes that take place in the relationship are equally challenging. Thus, these couples may need to clarify their legal, financial, and social rights to effectively carry out their changing roles and responsibilities in relation to the partner with AD.

When Your Parent Has AD

If your mother or father has AD, it is natural for you to want to remain in your traditional role as son or daughter. It is difficult to change patterns of behavior with someone you have known your entire life. Expectations and ways of communicating tend to become entrenched in long-lasting relationships—for better or for worse. For example, it may feel odd to act as the decision maker for someone who as a parent had authority over you at one time. But as unsettling as it may be at first, impairment in your parent's memory, judgment, language, orientation, and visual-spatial relations will require that you regularly give them direction, reminders, and other forms of help.

If your parent is widowed or divorced, you may be the one who ultimately assumes the leadership role. Does this mean that you are now in a position of "parenting your parent"? It is hard to avoid thinking of being in the leadership role in these terms. It is true that you may become responsible for meeting many of the emotional and practical needs of a parent with AD in ways that are similar to being a parent to a child. One son noted, "My dad has always been my mentor. It is hard to accept that he now needs me in the same way." Madeleine L'Engle describes this problem in her memoir about her mother with dementia: "I do not want power over my mother. I am her child; I want to be her child. Instead, I have to be her mother."[4] It is a mistake to think in terms of a complete role reversal for one inescapable reason: Your parent is and always will be your parent, and you will always be your parent's child. Also, children normally learn from their parents—but a person with AD will not always learn from you or remember your good intentions. Children also become less dependent over time, whereas the parent with AD will gradually become more dependent, in spite of your best efforts.

Although your parent's thinking and behavior may appear child-like at times, a person with AD is an older adult with a brain disease, not a child. Therefore, you must take into account your parent's unique personality and lifetime of experience. Parents typically fear any form of dependence on their children. Helping a parent with AD to retain a sense of freedom and avoid thinking of him- or herself as a burden is crucial in affirming his or her self-esteem.

How you cope with your parent's disease is likely to be influenced by your past relationship with him or her. If you enjoyed a good relationship, you at least have a solid foundation for growing into the role of leader. It can be extremely difficult to assume this key role but it can be done. Although this process will take time and practice, it will eventually feel more natural. One woman interviewed in the educational video, *From Here to Hope,* remarks, "It seemed that I was suddenly in the position of being Dad's lifeline. That was very awkward for both of us. It still has its awkward moments, but not nearly as many as in the beginning. We know each other a lot better now."[5]

However, even in the best parent-child relationship, it is very easy for you as the son or daughter to slip back into feeling like a beleaguered adolescent now and then. The typical adolescent struggle for independence is often played out in conflict with one's parent. If a parent with AD questions your leadership role, the old relationship battles may seem to be erupting all over again. Hurt feelings from your childhood may be consciously or unconsciously awakened. One daughter described this dilemma:

> My mother still has a knack for ticking me off whenever she tries to correct me or is critical of some decision. I feel like I'm sixteen-years-old again and that she doesn't trust me to make good choices. I guess the old tapes in my head get replayed in these situations. I forget that I am an accomplished forty-nine-year-old woman dealing with a seventy-seven-year-old woman with Alzheimer's who just happens to be my mother.

Remaining objective in the midst of emotionally charged encounters with your parent often requires the help of others. You may need your spouse, other relatives, friends, or a professional counselor to help you resolve your mixed feelings and achieve a mature outlook on your parent's disabling condition. Participating in a support group for adult children may also be useful.

If you did not have a good relationship with your parent or major issues from your past are still unresolved, you will definitely need help adapting to your changing role. Because of the nature of AD, it is now too late for you to settle any old differences with your parent on a one-to-one basis. Interpersonal conflict cannot continue without disastrous consequences for both of you. You must find other means of working out your problems with your parent, preferably through counseling. Meanwhile, you will need to call on others with whom you can share the leadership role. If you have a loving and supportive spouse, for example, he or she can often assume this role with less difficulty due to the absence of "emotional baggage" that you have in relation to your parent with AD. Without the benefit of such help, you may feel ill equipped to assume your new role. Your desire for relief, even escape, may be strong. Again, individual counseling and participation in a support group may be helpful.

You also cannot ignore that you have other priorities besides assuming leadership on behalf of your parent. Your marriage, children, and other relationships deserve attention, too. Your job and other interests may also demand your time and energy. The growing needs of your parent and these other personal responsibilities are bound to compete from time to time with your own needs. You will need to examine your priorities and perhaps scale back on other commitments to make room for the changes in your parent's life.

If you have brothers and sisters, it would be ideal if everyone in the family shared responsibilities equally and fairly on behalf of your parent with AD. In reality, however, one person usually ends up assuming the primary role as leader. If possible, the leader can delegate certain tasks to siblings. For instance, one of you can manage your parent's bills while another can take care of medical and dental appointments. Good communication is essential to maintain cooperation among all concerned. Old rivalries often emerge if siblings have not gotten along or worked well together in the past. It takes effort to put aside personal differences to serve the interests of the parent with AD.

Siblings who do not live nearby or who have infrequent contact with the parent with AD may not appreciate the extent of the problems associated with the disease, and they may not understand your growing responsibilities. Just as you had to overcome your initial doubts about the seriousness of the symptoms, your siblings may also need time and experience to face up to the facts. Although you may need to be assertive in making your expectations known, patience is also necessary in dealing with them. In their own time and way, your siblings may offer some measure of help. In the meantime, you may be accused of exaggerating the symptoms, promoting your parent's dependence, or seeking undue control over his or her decisions. Lack of experience, denial, and mistrust may motivate this type of thinking on the part of siblings, so you may need to exercise some extra patience. Keep in mind that you know things that they don't know or wish to know.

If you cannot persuade your doubting siblings to change their minds, it is best to call on a physician, nurse, social worker, geriatric care manager, or another helping professional to convene a family conference and lay out the facts. In this way, your motives are no longer at the center of the discussion. The focus shifts to your parent alone. An objective and knowledgeable outsider can educate others about the disease and your parent's need for care in ways that you cannot begin to address. A family conference can be a useful means of bringing all concerned to a common understanding. At the same time, your siblings may realize that you and your parent with AD have legitimate needs.

Being as inclusive as possible is essential for all concerned to make informed decisions about how each person will respond. If your siblings cannot attend such a conference in person, arrangements can often be made for them to join via a speakerphone or Web-based technology such as Skype. Or you may wish to arrange a separate phone discussion for a later time with those unable to attend the conference. You might also consider audiotaping or videotaping the conference. With your parent's written permission, you can also arrange for copies of his or her medical record to be sent to siblings who are unable to attend a family conference.

What About Kids?

The youngest family members may be affected by the challenges of caring for someone with AD, for better or worse. The interaction between young children and a great-grandparent, grandparent—or even a parent—who has AD, can be rewarding or distressing depending on the overall tone set by others in the family. Teenagers and younger children can have many positive effects on people with AD. Perhaps because they are less inhibited than adults, children can be quite accepting of someone with AD. Children can learn to engage someone with AD in ways that are mutually beneficial and enjoyable, sharing simple pleasures like taking a walk, tossing a ball, drawing a picture, putting together a puzzle, reading a book, dancing, singing, watching a video, or doing household chores. They can trigger fond memories and elicit nurturing instincts.

Generally, young children mirror the way in which their parents react to someone with AD. If a parent is irritable and impatient, a child will reflect these reactions. If a parent copes well and takes the time to explain the disease to a young child, then a good adjustment by the child can be expected, too. Relationships can become complicated when the person with the disease, typically a grandparent, lives in the household with a young child. The child may be at risk of receiving less attention as the focus of family life switches to the person with the disease. A child may act out dissatisfaction with the living arrangement by withdrawing from the family, doing poorly in school or with peers, or getting upset with the person with AD.

In such situations, steps need to be taken to ensure that teenagers and young children have opportunities for time, attention, and discussion with their parents. Otherwise, they may feel overwhelmed by the demands on them and the rest of the family. Their parents can reassure them that they have an important place in the family. Teenagers and even younger children can learn to share effectively in the care of people with AD. Children may respond well to their role as helpers. They may provide great enjoyment to the person with AD and learn valuable lessons about caring for others in the process. Fortunately, there are now lots of books and videos for teens and younger children to help them learn about AD and caring for someone with the disease. I highly recommend the HBO documentary that tells five stories of children, ages six to fifteen, who are coping with grandfathers or grandmothers with AD. This film, available for free viewing at www.hbo.com/alzheimers, is based on the book *What's Happening to Grandpa?* by Maria Shriver, whose father had AD.[6]

Telling Others About the Diagnosis

Just as you may have been reluctant to recognize the symptoms of AD or to accept the diagnosis at first, other family members, friends, and neighbors may not understand what is happening to the person with AD. They may lack the direct experience you have of seeing the symptoms unfold or hearing the diagnosis firsthand. They deserve to know the facts if their help is expected, otherwise they may become puzzled and troubled by the symptoms. Or, because of their lack of understanding, they could become frustrated in their attempts to get the person with AD to "act normal," for example, to remember certain things. Still others might be put off by the symptoms and then stop calling or visiting. If kept in the dark about the diagnosis, they are likely to find excuses to distance themselves. On the other hand, those who are informed of the diagnosis usually appreciate the explanation and may feel relieved to have an opportunity to be helpful. Unfortunately, some people do not handle the news well and eventually stop calling or visiting. Overall, however, others usually meet the diagnosis with acceptance and a desire to be helpful if given the chance.

Some people with AD and their loved ones may be adamantly opposed to telling anyone of the diagnosis outside of a small circle of close relatives and friends. They may unfortunately have a fear of being stigmatized and treated differently. One woman with AD noted, "My friends at the country club would drop me like a hot potato if they knew I had this problem." She also expressed worry that their help would make her feel like an "invalid." She added, "What they don't know won't hurt them." Another woman noted, "The last thing I want is sympathy, and that's what I always seem to get." Such worries are understandable, yet the reality is that most people already sense something is not right.

Those who spend little time with the person with AD may not see the degree of symptoms. In addition, people with the disease sometimes have an uncanny ability in the early stages to "rise to the occasion" and hide the symptoms. Physical appearances may be deceiving as well. In many respects, AD is an invisible disease in its early stages, since there are seldom any physical manifestations. The appearance of good health, coupled with social abilities, may give others the idea that nothing is wrong. In an educational video, *Alzheimer's Disease: Inside Looking Out*, a woman named Barb remarks, "Outwardly I look perfect, so usually nobody can tell anything is wrong. They don't notice what's happening with me. To me, succeeding with this disease was seeing how many people I could fool."[7] After explaining some of her own "cover-up strategies," Christine Boden writes in her story about living with AD, "After a social chat with you, when I might have seemed so incredibly well and mentally focused, I sink back exhausted, wrung out and empty of all showmanship. It may take me a few hours lying down with my eyes closed to recover."[8]

Casual observers may wonder if reports about the person with AD are untrue or exaggerated. They may have little or no knowledge about the early stages of the disease and think of it strictly in the dramatic terms often portrayed in the media. You and others close to the situation may be upset over these wrong impressions and the misunderstanding demonstrated by others. One woman expressed her dismay over the reactions of her husband's extended family to his disease: "His brothers and sisters see him only on major holidays and then they talk about old times together. Of course, they can see that he can reminisce so they assume his memory is fine. They have no idea what is happening with him day to day."

It can be confusing or upsetting for family and friends to be left uninformed about someone who has been diagnosed with AD. Keeping them in the dark can result in gossip, rumors, resentment, avoidance, and other unpleasant consequences. It can also be difficult for you to maintain a façade and keep the diagnosis a secret. It is not realistic to always keep the person with AD out of the way of people and situations that might expose her or his difficulties. And as the disease progresses, it will become harder to explain away the symptoms.

The husband and son of the woman quoted earlier (who wanted no one at her country club to know about her diagnosis) admitted growing tired of making excuses for her, although they wished to honor her request. They noted that several friends had expressed concern about her state of mind. She grew less adept at hiding her symptoms as her disease advanced. In addition, her husband felt isolated because he could not discuss their situation with others. Eventually, he was able to reveal her diagnosis to their circle of friends, thus gaining a new source of help and understanding. A few people could not handle the news and drifted away. The husband reasoned that they were not true friends after all.

As with most issues confronting you in your role as leader, the decision about disclosing the diagnosis must be weighed in light of the needs of the person with AD and the needs of others, including yourself. Protecting privacy and upholding secrecy about the diagnosis eventually proves unrealistic. At some point you will have to break the silence and let others learn the truth. They can then choose for themselves whether to become involved in some way. If there is a long delay in spreading the news, most people figure out the truth anyway. How and when this news is revealed is also a personal decision. Sometimes it is first done one-on-one with selected relatives and friends. You can also make an announcement by sending a letter to everyone the affected person knows. Such news should begin with the medical facts, especially the current symptoms and needs of the person with AD. There should also be an explanation of how others might be helpful both now and in the future. Finally, the importance of maintaining a caring attitude toward the person should be stressed in disclosing the diagnosis to others. The following sample letter illustrates how the news might be shared with others:

Dear family and friends,

I am writing with some news about my dad and a request for your help. Over the past few years there have been gradual changes in his memory and thinking, so we recently took him to a doctor for a medical evaluation. After conducting several tests, the doctor explained to our immediate family, including Dad, that he has symptoms of Alzheimer's disease. We were shocked at first, but Dad seemed unfazed by the diagnosis. We're told that the disease progresses slowly in most cases and that Dad may stay about the same for months, even years. We are hoping that the medication he is now taking will slow down the progression and partially improve his forgetfulness. There is no magic pill for Alzheimer's disease, but researchers are making strides in understanding its causes and developing better treatments.

Dad looks well and feels fine most of the time. Physical problems are not apparent at this stage. He does not seem as quick and talkative as he was in the past, although he still has a good sense of humor. He likes to talk about "old times," but his memory of recent events is getting poor. He enjoys people, but sometimes the fast pace of conversations or the commotion of younger kids bothers him so we try to accommodate him. He still drives a car but no longer ventures outside the local area for fear of getting lost. He enjoys playing golf but needs encouragement to do so, as he feels embarrassed that he forgets his score. He helps with all sorts of tasks but needs reminders along the way. Dad is remarkably "normal" in some ways and yet quite different from his "old self" in other ways.

Dad's disease has been difficult for all of us, especially our mother. Dad is no longer the man he was a few years ago, and this has caused Mom much grief, though she is coping relatively well. She has made many adjustments to his needs, and those of us who live nearby are doing our best to pitch in. The doctor warned us that Dad will need more of our time and energy as his symptoms worsen.

Mom and Dad clearly do not want pity, but they need to be in contact with supportive people. Your visits, outings, phone calls, cards, and letters would let them know that you care about them in this difficult time. Please call or write if you have any questions. I will occasionally update you about Dad's condition and his changing needs. Both Mom and Dad will need emotional support and practical help along the way. I hope that all of us can help them make the best of a difficult situation. Your concern is most appreciated.

Sincerely,
(Your name)

The Reactions of Others

It is difficult to predict how relatives, friends, neighbors, and others will react to the knowledge that someone close to them has a disabling brain disease. AD can have deep personal meaning for people, both real and symbolic. For some it evokes their fear of death; for others it is one of life's challenges to be confronted with grace and dignity. Just as your relationship with the person with AD is changing, your relationship with others must change, too, as new priorities arise. Some loyal people will stand by you; others may disappoint you with their seeming insensitivity. Some people will surprise you with their compassion, and others will sadly drift away.

You will need to surround yourself with as many people as possible who offer both practical help and emotional support. These relationships need to be appreciated and nurtured. One person may be capable of sharing a wide range of responsibilities, while another might manage an occasional bit of help. It is important for you to know who will really help you, and this requires that you make others aware of your needs. You cannot expect people to know what it is like to be a leader on behalf of someone with AD. Because few have had the kind of firsthand experience you have, they need clear instructions about how to be helpful both now and in the future. Your expectations need to be as explicit as possible.

If some close relationships prove disappointing, you need to evaluate how far you want to go in pursuing them. Some people may stop calling or visiting despite your requests for help. You may find it hard at first to understand their avoidance. It may be even harder to let go of your expectations. Nevertheless, pursuing those who cannot commit themselves can often cause much resentment and bitterness. It is better to focus your energy on more fruitful activities. Don't allow frustrations to dominate your life when you have such pressing priorities at hand. If possible, seek strength through forgiveness.

Some well-meaning people may give unsolicited advice or criticism about "what is best" for you and the person with the disease. They may suggest that you to try unproven remedies or advise you to do something different. Their seemingly good intentions may be overshadowed by their unwillingness to listen to what you really need. Encourage them to spend time with the person with AD to fully understand the complexity of the situation. Direct contact with the person with AD could mellow them and enable them to better understand your perspective. For example, you could invite them to spend an afternoon or weekend with the person with AD, and by the end you may have gained an ally.

Again, AD has a ripple effect on relationships. This starts at the center with the affected individual and spreads to that person's entire circle of family and friends. If you are closest to that center, you will naturally feel the effects of the disease most profoundly. As you gradually take charge of a loved one's life, your own lifestyle will change accordingly. Whether this proves to be a positive or negative experience for you will depend upon decisions you make along the way. This will require self-reflection, perhaps at a much deeper level than ever before in your life. A son reflects on his relationship with his mother with AD:

> What we are going to discover here is as much about ourselves as it is about the one who has Alzheimer's disease. Our relationship with one another is changed now, but it is not yet ended. There is for us an opening, an opportunity that will be our last chance together. It can become a very meaningful new period in which we find new roles and finally come to terms with what our lives until now have meant.

A chronic illness can bring out the best and worst in relationships. Rather than focusing on the negative aspects, this can be a time for healing old tensions and strengthening bonds within your circle of family and friends. The real test of your courage often begins with making tough decisions about practical matters. I will address some key decisions in the next chapter.

7 Making Practical Decisions

Even if you are on the right track,
you will get run over if you just sit there.

Will Rogers

The changing nature of the relationship between you and the person with AD will often be reflected in the variety of decisions that now need to be made. Several areas of concern, typically involving safety, come to the fore in the early stages: driving a car, managing medications, maintaining a proper diet, and handling finances. For people who have AD and live alone, the ability to remain independent becomes questionable and issues related to their personal freedom may come up. There may be a clash between the preferences of the person with AD and your perceptions of his or her needs. You will need to be assertive in dealing with these practical matters, while remaining respectful of the other person's wishes. Keep in mind that any change in one's lifestyle requires memory and thinking skills that are diminished because of the disease. Resistance to change can be expected. However, if you do not adopt a proactive stance, a crisis may develop. There may be negative consequences if you do not act in advance of preventable problems.

Ensuring Safety on the Road

Perhaps no issue raises as much dispute as the ability of the person with AD to safely drive a motor vehicle. In our culture, driving is more than a means of transportation and staying connected to other people and places. It is also a symbol of personal freedom. Getting a driver's license is considered a rite of passage into adulthood, as is taking ownership of your first car. Thus, driving a motor vehicle has both practical and emotional implications for all drivers. But driving is not a personal right, no matter how important it may be to one's lifestyle. It is a privilege regulated in accordance with certain standards of competence, and safe driving is a paramount concern, given the potential for injury and death from crashes. Unfortunately, the driving ability of a person with AD is often compromised early in the disease. On the other hand, some people with AD retain good driving skills for months, even years, in spite of their symptoms.

Driving a car safely requires the ability to quickly process lots of information. Brain functions for safe driving include judgment, coordination, orientation, concentration, memory, and visual-spatial skills. Impairment of any of these abilities may affect driving skills and lead to traffic violations and accidents. According a study published in the *Journal of the American Geriatrics Society,* the first driving skills to go are judgment, awareness of how one's driving affects other drivers, and speed control.[1] Other indicators that driving skills may be deteriorating include braking often or unexpectedly, not obeying traffic signs and signals, or veering from one's lane. These warning signs should not be ignored—the stakes are too high.

Several medical societies have weighed in on the issue of driving and AD but there is no clear consensus about when someone is unsafe to drive. What is clear is that as the disease worsens, the hazards increase, too. No standard tests are routinely used to assess if someone in the early stages of AD is too impaired to drive safely. In the end, it boils down to a judgment call. You may have to weigh in here, especially if the person with AD does not perceive a problem that is readily apparent to you or others. The individual's desire to continue driving may conflict with your concerns about his or her impaired driving skills.

Just as there is no medical consensus on this issue, there is no standard public policy in the United States or Canada in relation to drivers with AD. Most states and provinces require more frequent testing of older drivers than younger drivers, but this method is not foolproof in identifying unsafe drivers. Most state and provincial governments have Medical Review Boards that require drivers to provide notification of a medical condition that potentially compromises driving performance. For example, if someone is newly diagnosed with a seizure disorder, this condition is reportable. Although laws may not mention AD explicitly as a condition that poses hazards, the disease potentially fits into this category. Again, however, there is no clear medical or legal consensus to offer guidance.

At present, no state except California requires retesting of driving skills if someone has been diagnosed with AD. There is no question that the dangers of driving a car increase with the worsening of symptoms. As a result, the state of California no longer allows drivers in the middle and late stages of the disease, as measured by a screening test, to renew their driver's license. In most places, though, the decision to restrict or discontinue driving is done informally on a case-by-case basis. Public safety is often determined by a decision made by individuals.

In research studies, a driving simulator and a special road test have been shown to be fairly effective ways of assessing driving fitness among drivers with AD. On the other hand, this may not be a practical solution. A two-minute test involving an individual's ability to recognize ten common traffic signs has also been suggested as an easy means to determine the need for further assessment of driving skills. One major study found that deficits in visual-spatial skills were the best predictors of which people in the early stages of AD had driving problems. These skills relate to the ability to judge distances, maneuver correctly, and navigate in unfamiliar territory. Psychologists can use several standardized tests to assess visual-spatial skills. Other healthcare professionals have not yet adopted such tests as routine practice. The lack of medical or legal guidance on the issue of driving means that either the person with AD or others knowledgeable about his or her driving skills must make a decision when to restrict driving. While this individualized approach supports the liberty of each driver, it also poses a risk to public safety.

Fortunately, most drivers with AD adjust their driving practices to compensate for declining capabilities. They often reduce or stop driving after dark or in bad weather and avoid rush hour traffic, high-speed roads, and unfamiliar routes. Many voluntarily restrict their driving and eventually give up driving completely. They may fear getting lost, lack confidence in maneuvering a vehicle, forget rules of the road, or be inattentive to traffic. Sometimes getting a traffic citation or causing an accident shows them that driving has become too hazardous, but usually they are able to recognize their limits and act accordingly.

If a driver with AD is no longer safe on the road and does not readily recognize the risks, others need to point them out. Hearing your concerns about safety may be enough to convince the person to reconsider driving. Honest dialogue and negotiation often yield positive results. A frank yet diplomatic approach is recommended, in which you express your concerns and at the same time support your loved one's self-esteem. Giving up driving may not be a hassle if alternatives are available. Arranging for another driver or for public transit can ease the transition. If good transportation options do not exist for the person with AD or if their insight or judgment about safety is impaired, they are less likely to give up driving voluntarily.

Sometimes people with AD refuse to give up driving, although their skills are obviously impaired. For example, in the HBO documentary *The Memory Loss Tapes* a woman named Fannie who has AD is convinced that her driving skills are better than average, yet a road test reveals that she poses a serious threat to herself and others.[2] You may hesitate to intervene in such cases, rationalizing that the benefits of driving outweigh the risks. For example, a spouse who relies on the person with AD for transportation may see no alternative and deny the growing danger. In other cases, there may be concern that being told not to drive would be demeaning to the person with AD. Such personal considerations must be weighed against the more important risks to personal and public safety. To help you decide where you stand in this matter, here is a simple question to ask yourself: Would I feel comfortable letting a young child be a passenger with a driver who has AD?

If you believe that safety risks of driving do indeed outweigh the benefits, several solutions may need to be tried before the problem is resolved. Continued resistance by the person with AD, who has little or no insight into the dangers their driving presents, may require you to use increasingly stronger measures. In some extreme situations, even deception may be required. The following methods generally prove effective when you cannot reach a mutual understanding with an unsafe driver:

- Obtain the physician's cooperation in telling the person to stop driving. You will first need to privately share your concerns with the physician. If he or she agrees to accept an authoritative role, family members and friends are relieved of the pressure. Furthermore, a physician's involvement emphasizes that the decision is based on a medical assessment and not a subjective personal reaction. Since the person with AD may forget the physician's directive, it is helpful to have it written on a prescription or letterhead stationery. A note such as "Do *not* drive a car because of your medical condition" may be enough to settle the issue. You can use it later and direct any "blame" toward the physician. The physician does not have to specify AD as the reason; indicating a problem with coordination or vision may be more acceptable to the person with the disease. Most physicians are willing to assume this burden of responsibility if the dangers of driving are clear.

- If the physician questions your observations or the person with AD defies the physician's directive, consider a fallback position. Ask the physician to refer the person with AD to a local driver-evaluation program for a formal evaluation. Such programs are usually operated by hospitals specializing in rehabilitation. An expert, usually an occupational therapist or a psychologist with expertise in this area, will assess the person's driving skills using a variety of vision and cognitive tests as well as a road test. It is best if the road test is videotaped with a camcorder positioned in the backseat of the test car. In this way, the test can be reviewed later to illustrate any driving errors. A driving simulator may serve the same purpose. The expert's report to the physician should include recommendations about continuing, restricting, or stopping driving. Medicare and private insurance seldom provide reimbursement for a driving evaluation since in most cases it is not considered a medical necessity, so the customary cost of about $400 most likely will have to be borne privately. Such a driving evaluation may not be foolproof, but at least it offers a fairly objective way of assessing driving abilities.

- Ask the local police department to file a request for the person with AD to be retested by the Department of Motor Vehicles. If you explain the circumstances, police departments usually cooperate in the interest of public safety. Keep in mind that retesting does not always reveal problems encountered under normal driving conditions. Notify the company that insures the driver with AD and request that auto insurance be canceled on account of the safety risks posed by the disease. You probably need proper legal authority such as a power of attorney (see Chapter 9) in order to intervene at this level. Without auto insurance, the person with AD may stop driving for fear of being sued and financially ruined in the event of an accident.

- If the preceding steps fail, an option is to elicit the physician's help in revoking the driver's license of the person with AD. Physicians typically have the authority to initiate such action in light of certain medical conditions that pose driving risks, including AD. The physician can send a brief explanation of why the license should be revoked to the department of motor vehicles. A standardized form is usually available for such purposes. A medical review board or unit within the department of motor vehicles generally handles such matters, and you can expect quick action to be taken.

- In rare cases, a person with AD may continue driving after his or her driver's license has been revoked and the auto insurance canceled. A drastic option at this point is to make the motor vehicle inaccessible or unavailable. A mechanic can install a hidden starter button so that the person with AD cannot figure out how to start the vehicle. Disconnecting certain wires or switches can also disable the vehicle. Finally, getting rid of the vehicle may be the only way of resolving the problem.

For the most part, neither laws nor medical guidelines are clear about this important issue. Therefore, you are ultimately responsible for making an informed judgment that ensures the driving safety of the person with AD as well as the safety of the public.

Maintaining Good Health

A few health and safety issues also deserve close attention. These include making certain that the person with AD takes the proper medication and eats well-balanced meals. You need to carefully monitor these activities to prevent potential risks associated with misusing medications and having a poor diet.

Medications

Older people generally take many pills, both prescription drugs and over-the-counter products, including vitamin supplements and herbal medicines on a daily basis. Less than 15 percent of older people take no medications at all. Following directions to medications as prescribed requires a good memory. It is estimated that at least 25 percent of older adults fail to take the right dose or the right medication. Even if someone with AD is accustomed to taking medications at the same time every day, there is no guarantee that this routine will continue without a hitch, especially as the disease progresses. They may take too little or too much simply because of their inability to remember when they took the last dose. Failure to follow the correct regimen can have serious consequences, such as overdose, drug poisoning, or even death. Tens of thousands of people are hospitalized every year due to complications from mix-ups with their medications. People with AD who live alone are at the greatest risk for these kinds of problems.

To absolutely ensure that the person with AD is taking medication properly, you can follow one of two methods: Either observe him or her taking the pills or administer the pills yourself. A few other options also work, but they are less reliable. One is to count the number of pills remaining in a pill container and then figure out if the correct number has been taken since the last refill. If everything looks good, monitor the situation regularly. If you discover a problem, try some of these ideas:

- Keep written pill-taking instructions in a highly visible location or call the person on the phone to remind him or her about taking medications. Of course, these reminders may not work if the person with AD cannot complete tasks involving multiple steps.

- Arrange the medications in a weekly pill organizer and count the pills at the end of the day or each week. Keep the remaining medications out of sight.

- See if the pharmacy can provide medications in packs that enclose each pill in its own dated compartment. These "blister packs" are better than traditional amber-colored vials at keeping people up-to-date with their medications.

- Get a wristwatch or clock that beeps at designated times every day to remind the person with AD to take the next dose.

- Look into more sophisticated pill dispensers, which are available through medical supply stores, that use a timer and beeper to provide reminders. These dispensers are programmed to fit a person's medication schedule and are fairly simple to set up. Also look for computerized devices and other advances in technology that may be suitable for this particular need.

New, high-tech solutions are also available to assist with medication compliance including:

- GlowCaps, made by Vitality Inc., fit on most prescription bottles. A wireless chip causes the cap to pulse orange if the bottle isn't opened after a scheduled dose time. The caps cost $79.99 and have a monthly service fee.

- Rx Timer Cap LLC sells pill-bottle caps that count the hours and minutes since the container was last opened. The caps are offered free of charge by about one thousand participating pharmacies. They also sell online for $4.95.

- The MediSafe Project is a mobile application available as a free download in Google Play and the iTunes App Store. If a user misses a dose, the cloud-based MediSafe system alerts family, friends, and doctors.

Nutrition

People in the early stages of AD should have no trouble eating properly if someone is available to help plan and prepare regular meals. However, if the person with AD has been responsible for cooking their own meals, then some changes can be expected. Although she or he may still be able to prepare regular meals, the variety of foods and recipes usually diminishes over time. Often meals become simpler because of the difficulty of following all the steps necessary for large meals. Meal preparation may also taper off due to the risk of forgetting food left cooking and starting a fire. The person may skip meals or resort to small meals or snacks instead of maintaining a well-balanced diet. The effects of a poor diet may be disastrous for someone on a special diet, for diabetes for example, so it is vital that meals be monitored.

People with AD may also lack the know-how to shop for nutritious foods. They may have difficulty planning meals, organizing shopping lists, and handling money, and therefore they may end up buying less food. They may forget what's in the refrigerator and allow both fresh food and leftovers to become spoiled. Even if a person with AD buys the proper food, you cannot be sure that he or she will prepare or eat nutritious meals. You will need to check such details.

A person with AD may occasionally forget to eat unless reminded to do so. If someone else prepares a meal to be eaten later, the person may not eat it without a reminder. Some people with the disease lose their taste for everything except sweet foods. They may crave candy and other "junk food" that lacks nutritional value. Unwanted weight gain or weight loss, and, more seriously, malnutrition, may result from a poor diet. People with AD also risk becoming dehydrated or constipated if they do not consume sufficient amounts of liquids. Moreover, a poor diet can lead to other medical problems that may exacerbate the symptoms of AD. Here are a few ideas to help you ensure that someone maintains a healthy diet:

- First of all, aim to include the person with AD in decisions regarding his or her welfare whenever possible. You (or another family member or friend) might have to slowly take on responsibility for meal planning, food shopping, and perhaps even meal preparation. The person with AD should be encouraged to participate in these activities. Simplifying meals is a good idea, as long as the meals are nutritious.

- Home-delivered meals or Meals On Wheels are available in some cities and towns through senior nutrition programs. One hot meal and one cold meal are typically delivered directly to the person's home. Government programs may subsidize this service for those in financial need. Food preferences are not taken into account unless a physician orders a special diet, and the quality of food may not always be what is desired.

- Another government program called Golden Diners provides an inexpensive or free lunch as often as five days a week at senior centers, churches, and synagogues. These "nutrition sites" also offer opportunities for socialization. One drawback of this option is the need for transportation to and from the site.

Proper nutrition is essential for well-being. Problems like failing to eat or drink regularly or starting a fire while cooking can be disastrous. You must assess potential risks and develop creative solutions. If the risks are too great in your opinion, relocating the person with AD to a place where regular meals are provided may be the best option.

Other Safety Considerations

Some books focus a great deal of attention about potential dangers associated with AD that can result in harm. It is important be vigilant and take steps to promote safety in the early stages of the disease but it is not useful to be an alarmist and take precautions at every turn. No doubt as the disease progresses it will become necessary to take further precautions. For now, however, the basic safety issues addressed in this book are often the most concerning ones at this early stage. Nonetheless, two considerations pose danger at any stage of the disease:

power tools and firearms. Due to impairments in memory, thinking, and judgment, people with AD often cannot use these items properly. Therefore, he or she should not have easy access to either power tools or firearms, and, if they are to be used, supervision is always necessary. It is possible that the person with AD may resent restrictions that you impose. In such cases, it is useful to have a physician or another health-care provider support your decision and serve as a buffer. You may be able to prevent accidental injury and death by insisting upon supervision and restricted access to power tools and firearms.

Ensuring Financial Well-Being

Another major concern is managing the income and financial assets of the person with AD. People in the early stages usually give up on the complex tasks associated with handling money. Keeping things organized, paying bills on time, keeping track of investments, and making financial transactions are often too burdensome for them to handle alone. In fact, difficulty with performing calculations is often among the first signs of the disease. Making tax errors and forgetting to pay bills can have disastrous consequences, while exercising poor judgment in financial dealings can result in assets being drained. Therefore, you or another trusted individual might need to intervene by closely monitoring or taking charge of financial dealings. Exploring how to best help someone with AD manage finances should be done in the early stages instead of waiting for problems to occur later on.

People with AD may be at risk of financial exploitation by family members, friends, brokers, telemarketers, and other salespeople. In fact, financial exploitation is the leading cause of referrals to government agencies that are responsible for investigating allegations of elder abuse and neglect. Sadly, most financial exploitation is carried out against older adults by their close relatives who are rarely prosecuted for their criminal behavior. People with AD make for easy targets. They may be persuaded to write checks, hand out cash, give away credit card numbers, or transfer property to other people. They may then forget about such "gifts" or "investments." People with AD may also fall prey to variety of fraudulent schemes, phantom sweepstakes, sham charities, and "get-rich-quick" scams. In light of the enormous risks of involvement with such schemes, you should take steps to protect the income and assets of the person with AD as soon as possible. Some protective measures include the following:

- Do not hesitate to become involved if the person with AD asks for help with handling finances. Even if not asked, you should volunteer to help out to make sure that bills are paid on time and that assets are managed properly. The person with AD needs to formally appoint a trusted agent to act on his or her behalf. This does not mean that the person with AD is signing over his or her income and assets to another person, just the responsibility for financial management. Whether the appointed person will have partial or full responsibility will need to be negotiated. Various legal tools available for this purpose, such as powers of attorney and guardianship, will be explained further in Chapter 9.

- If possible, arrange for some or all bills and checks to be sent directly to you (or another trusted person). In this way, bills and income can be easily monitored. Again, cooperation of the person with AD will be needed to make this arrangement.

- Be alert to the fact that putting assets into *joint tenancy with right of survivorship* is a limited safeguard, since the person with AD technically retains access to the assets and has equal control. Moreover, joint ownership of savings accounts, real estate, and other forms of property has tax implications for both parties that must be considered. Eligibility for government benefits may also be negatively affected by adding someone's name to an account, title, or deed. A second type of property ownership known as *tenancy in common* may be a better option, in which each party owns a specified proportion and there is no right of survivorship. Either option should be carefully assessed in consultation with an expert.

- You can protect pension checks and other sources of income by electronically transferring funds directly into bank accounts. Another option is to arrange for a "representative payee" in which the person with AD formally authorizes someone else's name to be included on these checks. These mechanisms afford limited safeguards and comprehensive measures, such as power of attorney, are recommended.

- Become acquainted with a legal document called "Authorization for Release of Information for Fraud Prevention," that has been adopted by many states in the United States. This document is essentially a waiver of the right to privacy, which allows a bank to notify the bank customer and other named parties when it becomes aware of activity that is not consistent with the customer's usual banking patterns. Since bank employees are often the first to spot suspicious banking activity, they can help curb financial exploitation.

- To cut down on the amount of junk mail sent to the person with AD, get the person's name removed from mailing lists. To reduce the quantity of unsolicited mail and e-mail received from national mailing lists, go to www.dmachoice.org or make a written request to: Mail Preference Service, Direct Marketing Association, PO Box 643, Carmel, NY 10512. You can also ask the local post office to discontinue delivery of third-class mail.

- To cut down on telephone solicitations, register with the National Do Not Call Registry at www.donotcall.gov. This is a free service managed by the Federal Trade Commission, the consumer protection agency of the U.S. government. Also, you can easily block computer generated telemarketing calls with electronic products such as the TeleZapper, which costs less than $50.

- If you suspect someone is the victim of fraud, contact the local police department or the Office of the State's Attorney and the National Fraud Information Center at (800) 876-7060. Suspected cases of financial exploitation should be reported to the state agency on aging for further investigation; call (800) 677-1116 to get the phone number of your state agency.

Maintaining one's financial well-being can no longer be the sole responsibility of the person with AD. This responsibility requires that the individual remember and figure out too many details. You must intervene if the person with AD does not cede this responsibility. A slow, respectful approach by you is more likely to work than a heavy hand.

Alternative Living Situations for the Person with AD

It is estimated that one out of every five people with AD live alone.[3] Whereas they were capable of managing independently in the past, their self-care skills are under threat by the disease. Without considerable help from others, living alone under the cloud of AD can often lead to trouble. A person with AD is unfortunately prone to neglect oneself and to experience loneliness, fear, confusion, and other health and safety problems unless supportive services are put in place. You will need to assess the situation, identify any unmet needs, and devise a plan of action. Enlisting the help of others with these steps is a good practice. Involving the person with AD in the plan is also desirable but may not always be realistic. However, the goal should be to minimize risks while enabling the highest possible level of independence.

If the person with AD lives alone and receives no regular help, supportive services are strongly encouraged for the sake of safety, companionship, and convenience. Occasional assistance from relatives, neighbors, and friends invariably leaves gaps in the support required. Therefore, hiring someone to assist the person, moving the person into a relative's home, or relocating him or her to an assisted-living facility may be desirable. Such home-based services or other living arrangements are obvious considerations for many good reasons, but it is important to weigh all the advantages and disadvantages for everyone concerned. Clearly, the person with AD will be unable to live alone without increasing levels of help as the disease advances. The timeline for implementing changes, however, depends on each person's unique situation.

The preferences of the person with AD living alone should *not* be the paramount consideration in any decisions you make about his or her living situation. Your needs as well as the concerns of others are vital parts of the decision-making process. Those with AD generally prefer familiar people, places, and routines. Therefore, having a helper in the home or moving to a new place may feel threatening. Some people with the disease may feel demeaned or worry that helpers, no matter how well-meaning or useful, will take away their personal freedom. Allowing someone to come into the home is a big adjustment, and it may take several weeks before there is some measure of comfort with the new situation. Yet it is possible to introduce help casually in ways that ease the transition and improve the overall quality of the affected person's life. In some cases, the person with AD may gladly receive help with certain tasks and enjoy the company of a paid companion.

Some people with AD can remain in their own home indefinitely with proper help. However, a great deal of supervision may be needed to ensure that paid and unpaid helpers are addressing the person's needs. Part-time, full-time, or live-in companions are not always reliable, trustworthy, or helpful. Although good helpers may prove invaluable in allowing the person with AD to live at home, remaining at home may not always be the best option for a variety of reasons. I will address this topic in more depth in Chapter 9.

If part-time or live-in help is not feasible, relocation may be necessary. Despite the risks of having a person with AD remain in his or her own home, the decision to relocate has many drawbacks that need careful consideration. The person with AD may see his or her home as a safe haven, while other places may feel foreign and confusing. Anything new or different may feel threatening, since new memories must be created, which is a problem at the core of the disease. Finding his or her way around a new home can prove overwhelming for someone with the disease. Indeed, being uprooted and having to get accustomed to another home may exacerbate impairments in memory and orientation, at least in the short term. Moving somewhere else involves a series of big adjustments. The person with AD who lives alone may resist any type of change at first. You—and others—may have to move ahead with the person's best interests in mind and hope that his or her resistance eventually wanes. It helps to limit the person's participation in the details of any major change. It is important to note that if you plan and carry out all the tasks necessary to bring about needed changes, you can become exhausted. Therefore, be sure to enlist the help of others in this demanding work. If you are employed, you may be eligible to take job-protected, unpaid leave to handle these personal affairs; ask your employer about the Family and Medical Leave Act (described in Chapter 9).

If you do not live near your loved one with AD, you will need to do many things to ensure that all of her or his needs are met. Caring for someone with AD from afar can be a complex, time-consuming, and expensive endeavor. However, it can be done successfully if the proper people and services are put in place. Professionals known as "geriatric care managers," usually with backgrounds in social work or nursing, may be helpful in assessing needs. Care managers can also be paid to coordinate and monitor services if no one else is able to do so. For further information about care managers, the National Association of Professional Geriatric Care Managers (520-881-8008; www.care manager.org) offers referrals to its members throughout the United States. Because of the great investment of time, energy, and money involved in caring from afar, relocating the person with AD should also be seriously considered.

In the final analysis, you must serve as the judge in all these important matters regarding the well-being of the person with AD. Input by the person with AD on decisions directly affecting her or his life is clearly important. You may find advice and information offered by others useful in making the necessary decisions, and all the angles should be examined before putting a plan in place. Make it your business to find a trusted and experienced advisor—a friend or a professional—to help you navigate these decisions. Fortunately, few situations call for an immediate course of action, so you will have time to consider the options. Nevertheless, it is a good idea to have a plan in the works well before the situation becomes critical.

Doing the Right Thing

Although some people with AD gladly accept direction and assistance, others resist any form of help. Most people with AD retain an interest in doing whatever possible to have a say in their own affairs, including such matters as driving, medications, nutrition, finances, and living situation. One woman with AD made known her desire for autonomy in this way: "I'm not a loaf of bread that you can pick up and put here or there. We will talk about it, and I will listen so that I can make an informed decision—my decision." The opinions of the person with AD need to be considered whenever possible. Their remaining abilities should be tapped to the maximum feasible extent. For example, someone who is no longer able to cook safely may help with meal preparation under someone's direction. Someone no longer able to handle paying bills alone may still sign checks while another person handles the other steps. Such measures to preserve independence and dignity are part of this new dance—moving in and stepping back as needed.

Unfortunately, people with AD cannot always have the final word about key decisions. The disease may impair their judgment, sometimes resulting in an overestimation of their abilities, so that other people must sometimes decide what is in their best interest. In some cases, it is a frightening prospect to the person with the disease to trust others with so much authority over his life. Likewise, it is an awesome role for you to assume such responsibility for another person's wellbeing. However, you can be satisfied knowing that you are acting to protect the person with AD from certain risks and to ensure his quality of life. The person with AD may also feel relieved and grateful that someone else has taken charge of matters that have become difficult to handle independently.

It is easy to rationalize that someone you know, who ordinarily acted responsibly in the past, will continue to act responsibly in spite of having AD. Thus, the normal tendency is for you to overlook the person's difficulties with driving, money management, and other important matters at first. However, overestimating the abilities of the person with AD can present real dangers. In her memoir about her husband with AD, *He Used to Be Somebody*, Bigtree Murphy describes her reluctance to assume a leadership role:

> I was forced to accept responsibility for Tom's life, something I had fought doing under the premise that I was preserving his dignity. There is no dignity in forcing them to make decisions when they

no longer can. It took five years of our marriage before I realized the decisions were no longer his decisions, or our decisions, the decisions were mine. The relief that I felt when I finally accepted the task at hand as mine cannot be put into words.[4]

Weighing the potential risks against the person's autonomy is a tough job. Making the right decision on someone else's behalf can be difficult if the choices seem unclear. Enlisting others' help to objectively assess each decision may help clarify these choices and identify alternatives. A daughter described her decision-making process in relation to her mother with AD:

> I knew there was a chance that she might get lost or get into an accident while driving her car. But I was willing to accept those risks considering that she would be isolated from friends and family if she could no longer drive. Then, again, when I later saw that she might be losing her driving skills, I asked her neighbors for their opinions about her driving. With this extra information and some advice from her doctor, it was decided safety was at stake, and other transportation arrangements had to be made.

Disagreements may occur between you, others, and the person with the disease about the decisions you make. Advice and support from others are essential for keeping a proper perspective. Knowing how and when to exercise leadership on behalf of the person with AD is a delicate matter. At times, it may be readily apparent that it is appropriate to intervene, especially in dangerous situations. At other times, the choice may not be so clear-cut. In the end, however, it is you, as the person's leader and protector, who must ultimately make the distinction between acceptable and unacceptable risks.

Do not be afraid to assert yourself in this important role. Trust in your goal to do what you think is best for your loved one with AD. Learning to communicate effectively with the person who has AD will be useful in guiding your decisions. You will need to develop new skills for talking with and listening to someone whose communication abilities are faltering. In the next chapter, I address this topic.

8 Improving Communication

The single biggest problem in communication is the illusion that it has taken place.

George Bernard Shaw

In general terms, communication refers to the sending and receiving of messages. Good communication implies that both parties in an exchange share equal responsibility for sending and receiving messages. For example, if you speak to me, you expect me to listen, and vice versa. Many of the abilities that are required in good communication are diminished by AD. Although speaking and listening may appear to be relatively simple tasks, they rely on complex brain functions that become damaged in the course of the disease. First, an idea must be generated or organized. Second, it must be expressed, verbally or nonverbally. Finally, the idea must be received or comprehended by another person. These few steps require memory, language, perception, judgment, and the ability to process information quickly, yet one or all of these brain functions may be impaired in the early stages of AD. In this chapter, I will first describe a variety of communication problems that arise in the early stages of the disease and then explain ways of addressing these problems.

Communication Difficulties

A great deal of human interaction depends on our ability to remember new information and to share experiences. If learning is no longer easy due to the brain's inability to store new facts, communication becomes a daily challenge. People with AD usually make strenuous efforts to meet this challenge but fall short, no matter how hard they try. Because of the related frustration and embarrassment, they may avoid circumstances that will reveal their communication difficulties. They often become wary of social situations that are too mentally taxing. The burden of helping them falls to others who have the capacity to change the ways in which they communicate. In *Dementia Reconsidered: The Person Comes First,* psychologist Tom Kitwood uses a sports analogy to describe the role of the leader in communicating with someone who has AD:

> It is like being a rather resourceful tennis coach, keeping a rally going with a novice; whatever shot is attempted, provided it goes over the net, the coach will create something from it, and make a return that can enable the rally to continue. The coach needs attitudes and skills very different from those required to win a game with a player of the same standard; but this kind of play can be creative, demanding, and intensely satisfying.[1]

The analogy to a tennis coach suggests that you will need to hone or learn some skills in order to compensate for the communication problems posed by AD. Taking on this coaching role may feel awkward at first, but it is essential to keep the relationship on the right track. Better yet, having several "coaches" who support one another in this learning process can help create a healthy social environment for all concerned.

In general, someone in the early stages of AD is usually able to communicate effectively, as long as others provide some help. Some communication problems, or difficulties, that may occur in the early stages of the disease are:

- finding the right words
- comprehending abstract language
- talking on the telephone
- solving problems
- filtering out sights and sounds

- repeating questions or statements
- digressing, getting off track

Finding the Right Words

Although they might still be able to form complete sentences and to think logically, many people in the early stages of AD have difficulty finding the right words while in a conversation or remembering the correct name of an object or person. The overall richness of their vocabulary may diminish, and they may resort to using stock phrases or words to cover up—phrases like, "It beats me!" or, "Can't say as I do." They may also substitute general terms for specific words, saying, "I want to go to the prayer place" when they mean a church, or referring to their "money thing" instead of wallet or purse. Some people in the early stages use words such as *thingamajig* or *whatchamacallit*. They may also substitute related words, such as "coffee" for "tea" or "sugar" for "salt." Their difficulty with naming objects or finding the correct word may lead to long pauses between words and thoughts, which can prove exasperating for the other party in conversation.

A man with AD spoke of this difficulty: "The main problem is that I start to say something, and suddenly I don't know what I'm saying. I don't know how to say it, and whatever I was going to say is gone. The subject matter, the means of communication, the words I'm about to use next—they disappear. It's nerve-wracking."

A woman with AD offers a way in which others can help:

> There are times when I cannot find the right word. It simply disappears. If I let my mind go blank, it will often come to me. Sometimes I will lose my train of thought altogether. When I'm asked a question, it may take a while to organize my answer. If I am given the chance to collect my thoughts, I can usually have a fairly normal conversation.

In addition, people with AD who acquired a second or third language after childhood may become less fluent in these languages. They may gradually revert to their first language, since it is ingrained in their long-term memory. A man noticed this change in his mother:

"She emigrated to America from Poland at the age of thirteen. She became fluent in English within a few years and then spoke Polish occasionally. But now she is using Polish words more often, and her fluency with English is diminishing. That's becoming a problem for me because I don't know Polish."

Comprehending Abstract Language

Although people in the early stages of AD are able to understand concrete words and thoughts, they are likely to have trouble with abstract language. Figures of speech, slang, proverbs, idioms, sarcasm, innuendoes, jokes, and homonyms may variously be difficult for them to understand. Likewise, using pronouns such as *him* or *his* instead of referring to someone by name may be confusing. The person with AD may find it difficult to keep track of conversations, especially those filled with details that may be hard to remember. Above all, people with AD need to be given much more time than the average person to respond to a question because of difficulty processing spoken words and formulating an immediate response. A woman with AD remarked, "My brain is slowing down. It's like I used to have eight cylinders working easily in my head but now I am missing a few. I need lots of time to listen and respond to other people." Such difficulty in keeping up with conversations was described by Robert Davis in *My Journey into Alzheimer's Disease*:

> In my present condition, just seven months since diagnosis, there are times when I feel normal. At other times I cannot follow what is going on around me; as the conversation whips too fast from person to person before I have processed one comment, the thread has moved to another person or another topic, and I am left isolated from the action—alone in a crowd. If I press myself with greatest concentration to keep up, I feel as though something short-circuits in my brain.[2]

The problem of being outpaced by the seemingly rapid speech of others appears to be a common experience among people with AD. In *A View from Within*, Thaddeus Raushi describes coping with this problem: "Sometimes I just have to step back, get my mind off everything, and relax for a few moments after a conversation. I often find myself taking a deep breath such as the kind that follows an emotional event or tear-filled event. There is a period of recovery."[3]

Talking on the Telephone

Related to the difficulty with comprehension are several difficulties with using a telephone. Face-to-face conversations offer many nonverbal, visual messages, but talking on the telephone involves decoding the speech of others without the benefit of such helpful information. Christine Boden noted in her memoir about living with AD, "It's hard for me sometimes to understand what people are saying to me because I miss the first word or so and cannot make sense of the rest of the sentence. This is particularly true on the phone, where there are no visual clues or a context to help me try to work out what the topic is." Modern technology that allows for simultaneous video and voice conversation can ease this problem, including free or low-cost products available from companies such as Google, Skype, Apple, and Tango.

A related problem is that telephone numbers may not be recalled or found in a phone book or contact list. Although some phones can be programmed for "speed dialing" pre-assigned numbers, this feature may require memory and thinking skills hampered by AD. Another potential problem is remembering or writing down messages over the telephone. It is no wonder that most people with AD shy away from communicating by telephone. One young man described his initial misunderstanding of his mother's abrupt manner on the phone: "When I would call her, she would use every excuse to cut short our conversations. I thought that she was irritated with me for some reason. It took me a while to catch on to the fact that she could not tolerate the confusion involved with talking on the phone."

Solving Problems

Everyday life can become a series of problems for people with AD. At one time they were able to perform the simple tasks of life, such as driving and cooking, automatically, almost without thinking. However, since the disease disrupts normal thinking and behavior, customary ways of problem solving become less familiar and confusing. At the same time, others' expectations may not have changed, leading to misunderstanding and conflict.

As high school students, we learned how to solve geometry problems using the Pythagorean theorem ($A^2 + B^2 = C^2$), but most of us forgot this formula. Although we could once use this formula with relative ease, we can no longer remember it since there is no regular need to use it. Because it is no longer part of our problem-solving repertoire, we have simply relegated it to the brain's "trivia bin." For those with AD, the skills for solving problems are like trying to remember that old geometry formula. They experience frustration, particularly if someone else is not on hand to provide reminders or direction.

Imagine how frustrating it might be to once have had mastery over simple problems and now face increasing difficulty due to AD. Apart from these practical problems is the potential loss of self-esteem.

Filtering Out Sights and Sounds

Excessive stimulation of the senses due to too many competing sights and sounds may trigger confusion in people with AD. This "sensory overload" may then further complicate communication with them. They may cope poorly with too many people, too much noise, too much visual input, or too many activities. They may feel overwhelmed by too much information at the same time. It is as if the brain can no longer filter stimuli adequately. Consequently, it becomes saturated and cannot take in any more information, just as heavy rainfall causes flooding when the earth cannot hold any more water. Quite naturally, someone with AD may withdraw or become upset by situations that they find overstimulating.

The amount of stimulation that people with AD can tolerate may be in sharp contrast with their past ability. It may be difficult for others to realize just how little stimulation it takes for someone with AD to become mentally tired. On the other hand, this does not mean that all stimuli should be radically reduced or eliminated. Little or no stimulation can also breed boredom, anxiety, and/or depression. Rather, the proper balance of stimulation that can be well tolerated must be found for each individual. The following two personal accounts highlight the complications of sensory overload.

Robert Davis describes one harrowing experience while visiting a theme park at Disney World with his family. His resulting exhaustion led to a sudden worsening of his memory and language that lasted for six days. He learned to be less adventurous and adds, "Fear and tension fill me before any new event, even a wonderful event. I have to stay close to home and have less mental and emotional stimulation if I am going to have a normal and peaceful life."[4]

Christine Boden also writes about preventing sensory overload:

> Waiting in the quiet area of the airport, I am reveling in the new-found joy of earplugs. I sit as if isolated from all around me, with all sounds muted, muffled, distant—feeling like a deep-sea diver—watching planes and trucks on the tarmac, as restful and hushed as if they were tropical fish. No more struggling to keep up with a busy, multitracked, conflicting, and confusing world.[5]

It seems clear that some situations may overwhelm people with AD with an assortment of confusing sights and sounds, and they may withdraw from such situations or avoid them altogether. On the other hand, you and others need to anticipate the possibility of sensory overload and take steps to reduce or completely prevent it. Otherwise, someone with AD may become confused, irritable, or withdrawn.

Repeating Questions or Statements

A rather common feature of AD is the tendency for the affected person to repeat the same question or statement many times. The repetitions may take place just minutes apart. The listener may wonder if the person is doing this on purpose to get attention, since it can be hard to imagine that anyone can forget things so quickly. Yet, each time, the person with AD believes she or he is asking it for the first time. Repetitive questions or statements can also be a compulsive way of trying to remember, ease anxiety, or become oriented to one's surroundings. As a result, instead of shying away from the phone, some people with AD resort to calling at all hours of the day or night with the same questions or concerns.

One woman recounted how her mother began to call her repeatedly:

> She was scheduled to see the doctor and would call me a dozen times a day about the appointment. She was so mixed up about the date that every day seemed to her like the appointment day. I lost my temper with her a few times and stopped answering the phone at times, too. She would call me late at night with the very same question: "When are you taking me to the doctor's office?" It was hard to imagine that she could be so forgetful within minutes after I had given her the same information.

Obviously, patience and understanding are needed in dealing with an affected person's repetitive questions. Determining if the repetitiveness stems from an unmet need may help. Distracting the person's attention from his or her pressing concern may also be effective.

Digressing

Digressing, getting off track, or talking in circles may also happen to people in the early stages of AD. Their attempts to communicate may sometimes seem like free association to the listener. Their speech may be imprecise, wordy, and repetitive. They may forget what had been said to them and fill conversations with irrelevant details as a way of compensating for their diminished vocabulary or poor concentration. One woman with AD described her difficulty this way:

> The first symptom that I noticed had to do with my responses to questions. People would ask me a question, and I would give them a quick answer, and invariably it was wrong. I would have to say, "Oh, I'm sorry; I meant this." The second response was always better than the first one. I used to be able to give instantaneous answers, but now I can't. It's like my train goes off the track at times.

Redefining Your Relationship

There is no single approach or set of rules that will facilitate communication between you and the person with AD. There is no right or wrong way to communicate—only the ways that work for your situation and the ways that do not. In the long run, it is probably more useful for you to consider how to maintain or improve your relationship with the person instead of focusing on specific ways of dealing with the symptoms of AD. In this sense, your attitude may be more important than any single technique. Communication between two people occurs within the context of a relationship. If mutual trust, respect, and acccptance exist between you and the affected person, then you have a good chance that efforts to communicate will be successful in spite of the problems caused by the disease.

Most people with AD have limited insight into the nature and severity of their impairments. Consequently, they may seem indifferent about their day-to-day needs and may lack appreciation for the helpful efforts of others. They may have little or no concern about the past or future and may generally focus on matters concerning "the here and now." AD not only impairs their ability to remember but also their ability to plan ahead.

For family and friends, however, the relationship is also experienced in light of the past, with a history of shared experiences and well-established ways of communication. It can be difficult for the loved ones of a person with AD to separate the past from the present and to adapt to the changes imposed by the disease. Your old patterns of behavior and thinking may linger, even if you are aware that you will need to develop new expectations of the changing relationship. Adapting to the needs of the person with AD means redefining the relationship and accepting another person's view of reality. At the heart of understanding the perspective of the person with AD is deep appreciation of the present moment. Family members and friends who gain this appreciation often describe it as a breakthrough in redefining the relationship. Three examples illustrate this kind of insight.

Patti Davis describes her awakening to this reality about her father with AD, President Ronald Reagan, in her memoir, *Angels Don't Die:*

> We were sitting outside on the patio, and I looked at my father.
> His eyes met mine, and what I saw there told me it only mattered

that we were there together. The past was somewhere behind us. It had no place right then…. There was no past, there was only that one glistening moment, and I thought, this is what it means to live in the present. I hooked onto him right then, like Wendy holding on to Peter Pan—I learned to fly over the past into the bright blue space that was right in front of me.[6]

Filmmaker Deborah Hoffman describes a "liberating" moment in *Complaints of a Dutiful Daughter,* a documentary film about her mother with AD:

> For the longest time I insisted upon truth and reality being important. So she would say it's April when it was really May. And I would say, "Oh no, it's May." And finally it dawned on me, "What does it matter?" First, she'll say, "It's May?" and then the next minute she won't remember that it's May anyhow. Second, what does it matter if she thinks it's April?[7]

One man was bewildered by his wife's inability to recognize her problems with memory, judgment, and language. She was well educated and highly intelligent, and in the past could be counted on to tackle virtually any problem. He tried in vain at first to make her remember things. He pointed out errors in her logic. Their relationship began to deteriorate. During a road trip one day she declared, "The sky is a beautiful shade of green today," and he scolded her for her mistaken choice of words. In response, she felt hurt and stopped speaking for the rest of the trip. He later felt guilty about this incident and talked to someone about his rational approach, which obviously was not helpful. He then adopted a new philosophy: "From now on I accept that she is always right no matter what she says or does." With his insight into her viewpoint, their disagreements eased, and their relationship improved. When she did or said something that was a bit "off," he would just "go along in order to get along." The next time she commented that the sky was a beautiful shade of green, he simply said, "The sky is indeed beautiful today." He finally could share the positive feelings she was trying to express rather than get hung up on her "wrong" words.

The common theme of the above scenarios concerns the willingness of friends and family to enter into the reality of the person with AD. At first glance it may seem irrational to adopt this way of thinking. Nevertheless, it is the only realistic way of connecting meaningfully with someone with the disease. It takes self-confidence, empathy, and flexibility to do this. Focusing on the present will improve the quality of life for everyone involved; whereas expecting the person with AD to act and think "normally" perpetuates everyone's frustration.

Some general principles of communication are helpful in any person-to-person exchange. However, they are even more important in communicating with someone who has AD. These principles rest on one key element: the willingness to listen carefully to the other person and to respond accordingly. This involves communicating beyond the superficial level of words and connecting at the level of the human spirit. This deeper level of communication values the other person's point of view over the exact meaning and content of their words. A "meeting of minds" is the objective—but the responsibility for bringing about this shared meaning falls on you. This form of communication takes skill and practice.

Ways of Listening to and Talking with a Person with AD

Here are eleven simple ideas that can help improve your communication—both listening and talking—with someone who has AD:

1. gain the person's attention
2. eliminate background noise
3. use nonverbal cues
4. maintain a calm tone
5. listen actively
6. encourage expression
7. encourage comprehension
8. distract as needed

9. provide reminders

10. help with problems

11. accept silence

Gain Attention

Greeting the person with AD by name and using a gentle touch are good ways of getting his or her attention. On the other hand, interrupting someone in the middle of a task or a conversation may confuse him or her, so it is best to wait until there are no distractions. Visual and hearing impairments are quite common among people over age sixty-five, and these can make it difficult for you to gain their attention and may therefore pose further barriers to good communication. Attending to these sensory deficits will improve the level of the affected person's attention and your overall success in exchanging messages. Getting the person new or updated eyeglasses or having cataracts removed may improve not just his or her vision but your overall communication, too. New digital hearing aids are a great improvement over the older types and can clearly improve an affected person's listening and talking skills.

Eliminate Background Noise

To gain someone's complete attention, it is necessary to eliminate or reduce distracting noises such as television, music, radio, or the voices of others. A one-on-one conversation in a quiet setting increases your chances of getting and maintaining the attention of someone with AD. One man noted: "My wife loved being around our little grandkids until she got this disease. Now she can barely stand them for more than a few minutes if they are wound up. She has to leave the room because of the confusing noise. I've made a point of trying to keep their noise to a minimum." And one woman said this about her husband with AD:

> I learned pretty quickly that he could not hold a conversation if the TV was going on at the same time, so I turned off the sound when we needed to talk. Then I could not figure out why he turned up the TV so loudly when others came into the house. I finally real-

ized that turning up the volume so high was his way of blocking out the sound of other people while he was watching TV.

Use Nonverbal Cues

Giving the person with AD visual cues, such as with props, facial expressions, and body language, is an important part of nonverbal communication. Looking directly at the person and smiling will help to gain and keep attention. A gentle touch on the arm or hand not only gets another's attention, as noted above, but also provides an immediate connection. All of these visual cues are helpful in reinforcing verbal messages. In fact, our nonverbal behaviors may be better than our words for communicating effectively.

Maintain a Calm Tone

A slow and relaxed tone of voice conveys patience to the person with the disease; a loud and hurried tone will prove confusing. Although the person with AD may not grasp the exact meaning of your words, the tone of your voice can speak volumes. For this reason, people with AD will often "mirror" your emotional state. For example, if you sound anxious during a conversation, you may trigger anxiety in the other person. Be aware of your attitudes and feelings, since you may unintentionally communicate them through the tone of your voice and the pace of your words.

Most of us talk quickly and incorporate many ideas into our statements and questions. A person with AD is likely to lose track of rapid speech and become confused. Even a seemingly normal rate of speech can move too quickly for someone with AD to decipher. For example, if you are familiar with another language but not fluent enough to keep pace with a native speaker of that language, then you will appreciate the chance to slow down the conversation. You should apply the same principle when speaking with someone with AD. Slowing the pace of your speech may require a conscious effort. One daughter observed, "I have to really slow down my pace of talking whenever I'm around my mother. Otherwise, I see her getting anxious or drifting off within a matter of seconds." At the same time, you do not want to sound condescending, as if you are talking to a young child.

Listen Actively

Too often we think of conversing as two people talking together, but it takes both a speaker and a listener. The words of someone with AD may not be as important as the thoughts and feelings he or she is trying to express. Accessing this deeper level of meaning through careful listening may be your key to understanding what is being said. One son points out: "At times I could not figure out what my father was saying because of his difficulty with finding the right words. But how he expressed himself gave me some clues that helped me connect with him." Taking the time to listen in this way takes great patience, but it usually yields many benefits. A woman noted the importance of good listening in relation to her husband with AD: "It has become too easy to discount his input because it's difficult to understand him. Invariably, I have found that listening patiently to his input will provide something I had not thought about in a given situation." Careful listening is an art that requires practice. One man used a handy formula for learning the art of listening to his wife with AD: "I now try to make a conscious effort to listen twice as much as I talk."

Encourage Expression

As discussed earlier, the person with AD may need to "talk around" a topic before finding the right word or phrase. You should help someone who is having this kind of difficulty by supplying the needed language. He or she will usually appreciate your help. Forcing someone to struggle for words is unfair and unnecessary. At the same time, it is also important to leave extra time for the person to process a thought or feeling before they come up with an appropriate response. It is tempting to speak for someone with AD, instead of helping along a halting conversation, but you should avoid interrupting. It is also helpful to keep a conversation on track, since the person with AD may tend to get lost in a flurry of words and thoughts. Finally, correcting mistakes and getting into a contest of wills are counterproductive interactions. It is pointless to argue. The topic should be changed immediately if this begins to happen. Otherwise, the person with AD may feel put down, become frustrated, and hesitate to get into another conversation.

Encourage Comprehension

When speaking to the person with AD, you need to make sure that what you say is comprehended. You cannot assume that communication is taking place just because the other person is nodding in agreement or giving a superficial response. Therefore, it is useful to structure a conversation by first introducing a topic and gradually filling in the specifics. By going from the general to the specific, the person with AD will be better able to link the context and the details. One son noted: "My father was always a quick study on any subject. It took a while for me to realize that he could no longer keep up with complex explanations. When I caught on and managed to explain something in simpler terms, he was able to understand."

Open-ended questions can be confusing to the person with AD. Questions requiring a simple "yes" or "no" answer or offering a limited number of responses are more likely to be understood. One man described a common scenario:

> Whenever we went to a restaurant together, my wife would look at the menu for the longest time. When asked about her food choice, she would defer to me and say, "I'll have what you are having." But if I asked her if she wanted one thing or the other, she could readily give me her own preference. There were far too many choices for her on the menu, so narrowing the options for her was helpful.

Limiting choices regarding food, clothes, or activities to just two or three items enables people with AD to make their personal wishes known and helps them preserve their status as adults.

Likewise, abstract ideas and long-winded explanations are bound to cause difficulties. Concrete language and short simple sentences are better understood. You should also avoid using analogies, proverbs, idioms, and figures of speech; use simpler terms instead. It takes intellectual depth to reach beyond the literal meaning of sayings such as "a rolling stone gathers no moss" or "people who live in glass houses shouldn't throw stones." It is also important to remember that when giving directions to someone with AD, saying something like "hop in the car," for example, may be taken literally and cause confusion. Try to use specific words as much as possible. For example, instead of saying, "Here it is," try saying, "Here is your hat." And, again, it may also be more helpful to refer to another person by name instead of using ambiguous pronouns. Repeating or rephrasing a question or statement may also provide needed clarification. Finally, every effort should be made to avoid asking the most threatening and useless question of all: "Don't you remember?"

Distract as Needed

When a person with AD asks questions or makes statements repetitively, diverting her or his attention to another topic or activity may break the cycle. Distraction may be as simple as going for a walk or sharing a snack. Asking the person to reminisce about the distant past can also be a pleasurable diversion.

Distraction is also a good way of calming the person with AD when he or she becomes angry with you or is frustrated by a difficult task. There is a good chance that she or he will forget about the unpleasant situation in a short time. It's fair game to take advantage of the person's memory problem in such situations!

Provide Reminders

In the early stages of AD, many people with the disease use written reminders to compensate for a faulty memory. Calendars and diaries can be good memory aids and should be encouraged if they have been used in the past. Some speech therapists recommend using "memory wallets" and "memory books" that contain personal facts and photos to recall information and promote conversation.[8] Posting notes in a conspicuous place can also be useful. However, such written reminders should be stopped if they become a source of confusion. After all, one must remember to use the memory aids and must remember the whereabouts of such reminders. One man found success in giving his wife with AD an index card every day on which he wrote down responses to her frequently asked questions. For example, if she asked, "What day is it today?" or "What are we doing today?" he told her to look for the answer on the card kept in her pocket. She eventually got into the habit of looking at these cards without any prompting.

Giving repeated cues and reminders to someone with AD may help ease their anxiety over forgetfulness. But keep in mind that repeated reminders about emotional situations could actually increase anxiety and provoke repeated questions about the topic. For example, telling someone with AD that minor surgery is scheduled a month from now is likely to cause alarm. Therefore, it is often better to wait until the last moment to give information about an upcoming event. One young woman observed:

> I had to give up preparing my mother for anything. She would constantly ask about some future activity as soon as I would mention it to her. I have learned to wait. I do not tell her about an event until the time I actually need her involvement. Now she is not nearly as repetitive as before I figured out this tactic.

Help with Problems

Rather than posing a loaded question, try offering solutions. For example, in introducing someone you might say, "Here's your nephew, John, and his wife, Sharon," instead of asking, "Do you remember their names?" Avoid quizzing whenever possible and instead provide the right information. Guessing games not only fail to work but can also add stress.

Although a person's ability to perform familiar tasks remains relatively intact in the early stages of AD, at times any task, even a simple one, can appear too complex and demanding. For example, writing and sending a letter may involve as many as a hundred steps, and someone with AD may find it impossible to complete all of these steps independently. However, breaking tasks into small, concrete steps, giving reminders in the process, and assisting with difficult steps may allow for the person to complete the entire task. Again, patience and a willingness to slow your usual pace of doing things are required to lend this kind of support.

A new or unfamiliar task may pose a real problem-solving challenge to someone with AD. It may be akin to learning a new language in adulthood. One woman explained her futile attempt to simplify her mother's life:

I noticed that she had not been eating properly. So I bought her a microwave oven so she could cook food without a hassle. She never used it, complaining that she could not figure out the instructions. I never imagined that it would be difficult for her. On second thought, she had never used anything but a stove for cooking in the past.

Encouraging the use of remaining abilities involving familiar tasks will result in greater opportunities for the person with AD to succeed and be as independent as possible. For example, someone with AD may still enjoy playing familiar tunes on a piano but will not be able to learn a new song.

Accept Silence

People with AD tend to rely less on words for communication as the disease progresses over time. Nonverbal means of communication take on increasing importance. Someone with AD may no longer initiate conversations but may readily respond to questions from and comments by others. The normal give-and-take of interaction that adults enjoy usually changes in such a way that the person with AD settles into a quieter role. It can be a mistake to interpret this new-found silence as a sign of anger or depression. You may have more of a problem with this silence than the quiet person does. There is not necessarily anything wrong with your relationship, despite the decrease in the quantity and quality of verbal exchanges. And just because the person with AD does not talk as much as he or she did in the past does not mean that thoughts and feelings are absent. Either you can help the person express those thoughts and feelings or learn to accept the silence.

Whose Problem Is It?

The communication difficulties associated with AD illustrate why others must take an active role in preserving abilities and compensating for the inabilities of people with AD. In a real sense, customary ways of relating to the world have become difficult for them. As a result, communication also becomes a problem. From the perspective of people with AD, we are the ones who are making life difficult.

We must begin by putting aside our preconceived notions about the importance of intellectual abilities and adjust our expectations to the needs of the person with AD. It then becomes possible for us to enter their realm and feel comfortable with the changing relationship. They may not be able to articulate their gratitude for this sensitivity to their needs, but the atmosphere of trust, understanding, and openness fostered by effective communication will make life better for everyone.

Communicating well with someone with AD involves a learning curve. It may take months, even years, before you become comfortable with using a new set of communication tools in your relationship. One man noted that he made progress in changing his ways when he began to filter his ideas and words to his wife "through the prism of Alzheimer's." A daughter described her transition to becoming "like an improvisational actor" in regard to her mother's twisted language and thoughts. A period of trial and error can be expected as you make this transition to a new way of communicating. After all, a major shift in roles is taking place in the relationship, and old habits of communication are hard to break.

Reflecting on your successes and failures is critical to your learning how to best communicate with someone with AD. In *Alzheimer's, a Love Story*, Ann Davidson shares a powerful insight on coping with her husband's disease, based on mistakes she had made:

> I've learned to track that flash of reaction between situation and upset, to discover my intervening thoughts. When Julian does something odd, I sometimes think, "Stupid man!" or "Oh, God, he's getting worse!" or "I'm going crazy." These thoughts flash through my brain, faster than I'm aware of them. But when I stop and tell myself, "The man I love has terrible memory problems" or, "He can't help it," I react differently and better feelings emerge. Replacing harsh statements with more helpful ones changes the way I feel. Events alone don't create bad feelings. What we think and tell ourselves causes a large part of our distress. I can't control what Julian says and does; I can control how I react.[9]

Communication difficulties caused by AD may pose the greatest challenge to your relationship with the person with the disease. As Davidson notes, these difficulties cannot be controlled, but your reactions to them can be. You can adapt and learn new ways of communicating that can help bridge the communication gap caused by the disease. Communication is also central in helping your loved one with AD plan for the future. The next chapter focuses attention on several steps you will need to initiate in preparation for the near and long-term future.

9 Helping a Person with Alzheimer's Disease Plan for the Future

Failing to plan is planning to fail.

Anonymous

At first, meeting the present and future needs of the person with AD may seem overwhelming. No question that enlisting the help of others is necessary to ease the burden of making important decisions. But for now, all that is required of you in planning for the future is putting a few matters in order. Short-term goals include addressing legal and financial affairs, rethinking the living situation, and finding the right professionals who can help you and others in the care of someone with AD. If you first focus on achieving these goals, then you are more likely to succeed in achieving other goals in the future.

Finding the Time

Even before you get into the details of planning for the short term, it is reasonable for you to ask, Where do I find the time to do everything? Even if you are retired, you had other activities that occupied your time and energy before AD entered the picture. If you are employed either full-time or part-time, it may be a real juggling act to balance your job and your personal life, including responsibilities with the person who has AD. It will certainly require a rearranging of your priorities. Little by little, you will need to make room in your life for attending to the details of another person's life. You should not assume that all of your leisure activities are dispensable, since they are needed to refresh you and help you maintain a healthy balance in your life. However, you will most likely need to cut down on some of the things that you do.

If you are employed and in a position to retire or scale back your work hours, explore those options. If, on the other hand, work is a good outlet for you, consider other ways of finding time for caring for someone with AD. Look for creative alternatives that put some flexibility into your work schedule. Instead of quitting work altogether or being absent regularly, you could explore the benefits of the Family and Medical Leave Act.[1]

The Family and Medical Leave Act is a U.S. law that requires employers with fifty or more employees to grant up to twelve weeks of unpaid leave a year for the care of a parent, spouse, or child with a serious health condition, among other specified reasons. AD fits the definition of a serious health condition covered under the law. When the leave is finished, an employer must reinstate you at the same or equivalent level of pay and status. The leave can be taken all at once or intermittently. For example, you may choose to reduce your work schedule from forty to thirty hours per week. In this way, you can extend your leave throughout the year. An employer may require you to use any or all accrued paid leave you are entitled to under your customary benefits package as part of the twelve-week allotment. Under the law, an employer must also continue your group health-insurance coverage under the same terms and conditions as if you had not taken leave. To be eligible for this leave you must have worked at a company for at least twelve months and have put in at least 1,250 hours before the leave. You also must submit a medical certification form regarding the nature of the illness and give up to thirty days' notice whenever possible. One woman took a four-month leave from her job to plan for her mother's move into a retirement community:

> The leave from work gave me time to devote to a thousand details—like arranging medical and dental appointments, choosing the right place with Mom, moving her into her new home, and selling her old one. It gave my mother someone to lean on during

this difficult transition. I had peace of mind knowing that I could step back into my job. The leave was a godsend.

Time is a precious commodity that should be managed carefully, given the myriad needs of someone with AD. A woman whose mother has AD notes, "I'm no longer responsible for just my own life. I'm now planning for two at all times. I've never had to be so efficient!" One man whose wife has AD explains that he applies his business skills to address this challenge: "I see her disease as a massive project. I line up the resources to help us succeed. I had to orient my schedule to that reality. Priorities now fall into place more easily." This is a good approach to take when you consider the time-consuming demands of the disease.

Legal Considerations

One of the first things to consider is having the person with AD formally designate someone to act on her or his behalf with respect to legal and financial decisions. Though adults ordinarily are legally presumed to possess sound decision-making capacity, the person with AD eventually loses this capacity. There is no simple, clear-cut test that can establish when this happens. You can assume, however, that at some point in the course of the disease, the person with AD will no longer have the memory, judgment, and problem-solving skills or the mental capacity to properly manage his or her health-care and financial affairs. Mental capacity basically refers to the ability to receive and understand information, evaluate options, and make an informed decision that is consistent with one's personal values. Proper legal and financial planning enables people with AD to choose a trustworthy person to act on their behalf in the future. Certain legal tools called "advance directives" should be used before the person with AD loses capacity. These direct an authorized representative to act on behalf of the person with AD in the future, should it become necessary.

It is essential for the person with AD to be proactive and complete the necessary legal documents as soon as possible. Waiting until later means risking the chance that the person with AD may no longer be capable of designating an agent. The agent's main responsibilities are to represent the stated preferences of the incapacitated person and guard against abuse or neglect with respect to health and financial affairs.

The most useful legal tool available to the person with AD is the power of attorney (POA). Since the POA ultimately concerns all decisions affecting one's welfare, it is a very powerful legal document. This tool is considered "durable" in that the POA remains in effect after the incapacity of the person with AD, whenever that occurs as specified in the document. The POA establishes a legal, private relationship between the person with AD (the "principal") and someone of his or her choosing (an "agent") who serves as a substitute decision maker. The designated agent is entrusted with great authority to fulfill someone else's stated wishes at a later date, so this person must be chosen wisely. Only if the agent violates this solemn oath through abuse or neglect can his or her authority be challenged and revoked. The POA requires that a second person be named as a "backup" in case the first agent is unwilling or unable to carry out the duties. Standard legal forms that lay out the terms of this agreement are readily available, but specific terms vary from state to state. These forms are usually available for purchase at office supply stores, and many local and state agencies on aging distribute them for free.

Two types of POA are available: one for health-care decisions and another for financial affairs. The POA for health care not only identifies an agent for all health-related decisions but also includes directions regarding life-sustaining treatments (for example, whether to use a mechanical ventilator or a feeding tube). Since people have varying opinions about using technology to artificially prolong life, the health-care POA makes known one's specific wishes and directs the agent to carry them out at a later date. Again, one or two alternate agents are also named to serve in a backup role if the first agent is unavailable. It is not necessary to have this type of POA document completed by an attorney. However, consultation with an attorney may be useful in clarifying any questions and addressing special needs. The POA for health care requires signatures of the principal and a couple of witnesses but usually does not require notarization.

A popular version of the POA for health care form is "The Five Wishes," which includes provisions for care and comfort that are not typically found in standard legal forms. This form is valid in forty-two U.S. states and is available in twenty-six different languages. Contact www.agingwithdignity.org or (800) 594-7437.

In contrast to a POA for health care, a living will is a legal document that pertains only to end-of-life decisions and not to all health decisions beyond the point of incapacity. In a living will, an assigned agent's authority is limited to making decisions only at the point of a person's terminal illness. Furthermore, some states do not include decisions regarding the use of feeding tubes in their living will laws. The drawbacks of a living will can best be addressed by means of the more comprehensive and useful POA for health care.

The POA for property gives authority to a designated agent over the management of personal property and finances. This means that the appointed representative is given virtually all control of an individual's income and assets. The POA for property is critical to planning for the future care of someone with AD, since it specifies who is to be responsible for using an individual's income and assets to pay for any future costs of care. However, the POA for property does not provide exact instructions as to how the agent is to use the assets and income on the person's behalf. Although legal forms are also available for this type of POA, standardized forms may be limited in the powers they address. It is advisable in most cases to consult an attorney in considering the far-reaching implications of this type of POA. Completion of the POA for property requires signatures by the principal and two witnesses as well as notarization.

A living trust is a legal tool that requires the expertise of an attorney to fully explain its benefits for estate- and tax-planning purposes. A trust consists of a written agreement and a funding mechanism whereby a person (the "grantor") gives a trustworthy person or a bank (the "trustee") the power to control his or her income and assets according to prescribed conditions. The trust agreement includes specific directions about how, for example, to provide for the care of the person with AD (the "beneficiary") by using funds transferred into a trust account. The living trust also stipulates how funds are to be distributed after death and can be a useful means of avoiding probate. Co-trustees and successor trustees can also be named in living trusts. A fee is involved in setting up and operating a living trust, so although a living trust has many advantages over the POA for property, its expense and complexity may be impediments to choosing this option. Wealthy people routinely use trusts for many reasons, including a reduction in estate taxes. However, they can be helpful with handling small estates and limited resources as well. You should seek the advice of an attorney to find out which legal tools best suit your situation.

Regardless of which legal tools you use to plan for incapacity, you will need to make decisions as soon as possible about advance directives. Waiting means risking the possibility that the person with AD will no longer have the capacity to be involved in the pertinent details of planning. If either you or your loved one has doubts about how to begin the planning process, certified financial planners and attorneys who specialize in the growing field of "elder law" can help.

Although it is vitally important to discuss advance directives with the person with AD, it is not advisable to promote the discussion by suggesting that his or her incapacity appears imminent. Scare tactics are not needed if you can communicate that planning of this kind is beneficial for everyone. After all, incapacity may happen to anyone at any time for any number of reasons. Present the idea to the person with AD as a means of choosing his or her own agent and ensuring that personal income and assets are protected. Put the person with AD at ease by explaining the need for planning in simple terms and by focusing on the person's right to exercise his or her autonomy right now. Present the planning as a positive step to protect rights and not as an admission that dependence on others will happen sooner or later. This discussion should take place in a casual atmosphere and on a one-on-one basis with the person who has AD, since discussing these kinds of details in a group setting often leads to confusion. It may be helpful to complete these forms together instead of focusing solely on the person with AD, since every adult should complete POA for both property and health care, regardless of one's health status.

It should be noted that if the person with AD is married, the spouse is not automatically considered the agent. It is best to sit down together and choose who should serve as each partner's agent or trustee in the future. If planning is done jointly, full cooperation by the person with AD is likely. An adult child who approaches this matter-of-factly with his or her parent is also likely to get through the process with a sense of relief for all concerned.

The value of putting these kinds of safeguards in place cannot be overstated. If the person with AD does not complete advance directives through a POA or a living trust, others may take advantage of the situation. There may be theft, fraud, and exploitation by unscrupulous people, including friends and relatives. Someone with AD who lives alone may be especially vulnerable. Your (or anybody else's) attempts to manage the affairs of the person with AD, even when done with the best intentions, can be challenged if no legal documents have been executed. Likewise, attempts to prevent financial mismanagement can be questioned if nobody has been given legal authority to act on behalf of the incapacitated person.

If advance directives are not in place before the person with AD becomes incapable of making decisions, the only remaining option is for you or another interested party to petition a probate court for guardianship or conservatorship. Guardianship involves a judge determining that the person with AD is indeed incapacitated, after medical evidence has been furnished, and appointing someone, known as a legal guardian or conservator, to act on behalf of that person. Sometimes a judge will appoint a trust department of a bank to manage a person's income and assets, particularly if there is a dispute among family members regarding who should be in charge of such affairs. Guardianship can be fairly straightforward but can also prove to be a lengthy, divisive, and expensive legal process. It can be avoided if legal and financial planning is completed early in the progression of the disease.

Adult children should be prepared to manage the financial affairs of a parent with AD in case the well parent dies first or becomes incapacitated. It is helpful for the well spouse and the adult children or others to jointly discuss contingencies and to collect facts about all sources of income and assets. Management of income and assets, as well as living trusts, wills, and powers of attorney, need to be reviewed *before* a crisis occurs. Countless problems may ensue without adequate preparation.

Elder law attorneys and certified financial planners may offer guidance on a variety of tools available for planning for the future. Two professional organizations that provide referrals to their members include the National Academy of Elder Law Attorneys (www.naela .org or 520-881-4005) and the Financial Planning Association (www .fpanet.org or 800-322-4237). Free information on legal issues can also be obtained from the public-interest law firm known as the National Senior Citizens Law Center (www.nsclc.org or 202-887-5280). Other licensed professionals such as social workers, psychologists, and counselors may help individuals and families sort out the emotional issues and mediate disputes that sometimes arise when care decisions and money are at stake.

Financing the Cost of Care

In considering legal and financial planning, it is important to consider the related issues of costs and insurance. Health-care insurance typically covers the costs of acute illnesses and some preventive services including hospitalization, outpatient tests, and physicians' fees. However, most costs associated with a chronic condition like AD, which can be staggering, are unfortunately not covered by health insurance. You may eventually need to hire an in-home care worker or use the services of an adult day center. Residential care including assisted living facilities and nursing homes, which cost $5,000–9,000 a month, may be a future option.

If your spouse has AD, you will have obligations concerning payment for her or his care. And although a legal obligation may not apply if your unmarried partner or parent has AD, you may feel morally or socially responsible for contributing to the cost of care. What are some of your options to pay for such care? The following are key areas to consider regarding financing the cost of care:

• income and assets
• tax deductions and credits

- Medicare and supplemental health insurance
- state and federal programs
- Medicaid
- long-term care insurance
- a reverse mortgage
- life insurance settlements

Income and Assets

The bulk of home care and residential care expenses are paid for privately, that is, out of one's own pocket. The income and assets of a person with AD, as well as the joint income and assets of a married couple, may be tapped and depleted by care-related expenses. If you are an adult child, your expectations about receiving an inheritance should be put aside in favor of the needs of the person with AD. Every type of income, asset, and expense must be reviewed and considered to pay for care. If possible, consult a certified financial planner for assistance with the planning process.

Many older individuals and couples who lived through the Great Depression developed a habit of saving or investing their money to prepare for the possibility of hard financial times. They may be reluctant to use their financial resources, fearing that even harder times may lie ahead. One woman noted:

> My husband and I have been saving for a rainy day. It's hard to believe that the rainy day has arrived now that he has Alzheimer's. My son says it's raining cats and dogs, so I might as well get used to paying for new priorities. I did not expect we would have to use our hard-earned money in this way. Who expects this disease? Dying quietly in your sleep without a painful or expensive illness is a fantasy.

While this woman was concerned for her husband's welfare, the possibility that she may need care in the future must also be considered. The needs of the so-called "well spouse" have to be factored into care decisions and financial planning.

Balancing the real and potential needs of one or two people both now and in the future is no easy task, so every aspect of financial worth must be examined. For example, the chief asset of older people is generally their home. They may have a fixed income but have substantial equity in their home. Federal law in the United States offers tax exclusion from the sale of a principal residence for people aged fifty-five or older for up to $250,000 for single individuals or $500,000 for married taxpayers filing a joint return. Liquidating this asset may be a good option for some people but not for others. The importance of obtaining sound financial advice cannot be stressed enough.

Since most Americans with AD are older individuals, they are likely to be receiving Social Security retirement benefits based on their own or their spouse's employment history. However, someone with AD not yet old enough to qualify for Social Security retirement benefits may also qualify for another government program—Social Security Disability Insurance. This is income for disabled and blind persons based on employment history. Such benefits derive from an insurance program paid for by all workers through payroll taxes. To qualify for these disability benefits, a person must have worked long enough and recently enough to be insured. An application for disability benefits should be filed with the local Social Security Administration office as soon as a diagnosis of AD is medically documented. Under a Compassionate Allowance program, people with AD and related disorders are supposed to have their disability applications fast-tracked so they can be approved for benefits within weeks. Benefits continue indefinitely regardless of age, since AD is considered a permanent disability. For people who do not meet the employment history requirements to qualify for disability benefits, another Social Security program called "Supplemental Security Income" provides monthly benefits to those who meet financial-need requirements.

Whether a source of income is a government entitlement program, a private pension, a stock dividend, or an annuity fund, someone needs to take charge to make sure that all benefits are being received on time and that they are being managed properly. Thus, someone needs to be appointed by the person with AD to serve as his or her agent in these financial affairs.

Tax Deductions and Credits

Taxpayers in the United States can claim itemized deductions for medical, maintenance, and personal care services to the extent that they exceed 7.5 percent of their adjusted gross income. Most states also offer medical tax deductions in their state income taxes. Deductions typically apply to an array of expenses for care provided at home or in a residential care facility. You must document the need for such services and keep records of all expenses and payments. Services may include those provided at home by paid workers or expenses incurred at an adult day center or a residential care facility. If itemized deductions do not apply, a tax credit for "household and dependent care" may be available if the person with AD resides with you. How tax laws affect you depends on your situation. It is strongly recommended that you seek advice from a tax professional to make sure that you get the benefits you deserve. The Internal Revenue Service may also be contacted at (800) 829-1040 for the following free publications regarding tax deductions: Medical and Dental Expenses (Publication 502) and Child and Dependent Care Expenses (Publication 503).[2]

Medicare and Supplemental Health Insurance

Medicare is the federal health insurance program for Americans aged sixty-five and older. People under age sixty-five are also eligible for Medicare after receiving Social Security disability benefits for twenty-four months. Unfortunately, you will not be able to count on Medicare for any help with chronic or long-term care, since it was created primarily to offset the costs of acute medical conditions. And Medicare does not pay for in-home care or residential care except under narrow conditions for a limited period of time. Medicare and private insurance policies generally do not cover the costs associated with the care of persons with AD or most other chronic diseases. Likewise, supplemental insurance policies and health plans offered by managed-care organizations do not cover the costs of chronic care. Attempts to expand Medicare coverage to pay the costs of caring for people with chronic diseases have proven politically and economically impossible. Modest legislative proposals have been introduced to offer additional tax credits and subsidies to offset the costs of chronic care to individuals and families. Whether these proposals will be enacted remains to be seen, although there appears to be growing recognition on the political scene that families with loved ones in need of ongoing care deserve financial support.

State and Federal Programs

In an increasing number of states, combined state and federal programs are subsidizing home-based care. Eligibility standards for these entitlement programs vary from state to state. Generally, by paying for services through designated home care agencies and adult day centers, they are intended to serve those with low incomes and assets as a means of preventing or postponing the more expensive nursing-home option. For further information about state programs and specific community resources, contact the Eldercare Locator Service at www.eldercare.gov or (800) 677-1116, and you will be directed to local agencies.

Medicaid

Middle-income Americans probably face the greatest challenge in financing the cost of caring for someone with AD, since their income and assets must be "spent down" in order to qualify for government entitlement programs. Essentially, the person with AD must become destitute in order to qualify for Medicaid, which pays the majority of costs for nursing-home care in the United States. However, if the person with AD is married, his or her well spouse has some legal protection against impoverishment. The protected level of personal assets and income for spouses varies from state to state, although the right to keep one's residence is guaranteed. Protecting your assets and income as well as transferring property to others can be complicated, so it is advisable to seek the professional advice of an elder law attorney. The state agency responsible for administering the Medicaid program should be contacted for information about eligibility requirements and protections against spousal impoverishment (www .medicaid.gov).

Long-Term-Care Insurance

Private insurance is available to cover the costs of long-term care, but relatively few people can afford these rather expensive policies. Although costly, long-term care insurance can prove to be a good investment. The downside is that it cannot be obtained *after* a diagnosis of AD has been made since the probability of using services is high. Nevertheless, a spouse may want to obtain coverage for him- or herself. Since there are pitfalls and advantages to long-term care insurance, it is a good idea to compare different policies. The independent testing organization *Consumer Reports* periodically rates these policies (www.consumerreports.org). Also, a free service known as the State Health Insurance Program (https://shiptalk.org), which is available in every U.S. state, offers phone and face-to-face counseling about Medicare and these private insurance policies. In general, since governmental and private insurance do not cover the costs associated with the care of people with AD, most people rely on their income, savings, and other assets to pay for needed services.

Reverse Mortgages

Another means of paying for long-term care that has grown in popularity over the past decade involves using your home equity through a "reverse mortgage." Reverse mortgages were conceived as a means to help people in or near retirement and with limited income use the money they have put into their home to pay off debts to cover basic monthly living expenses or pay for health care. If you purchased your home, you borrowed a large sum of money and then paid it back in monthly installments over a number of years. As a result of your mortgage, you built up equity. With a reverse mortgage, instead of you making monthly payments to a lender, the lender makes payments to the borrower. A reverse mortgage is a loan available to people over sixty-two years of age that enables a borrower to convert part of the equity in their home into cash.

A reverse mortgage does not restrict how a borrower uses the proceeds. As long as you live in the home, you are not required to make any monthly payments toward the loan balance, but you must remain current on your tax and insurance payments. The reverse mortgage, which is a loan paid to you in monthly installments or in one lump sum, is not considered taxable income. Your home's value, your age, and the current interest rates determine the total amount of the loan. The older you are, the larger the monthly checks or lump sum, since your life expectancy is shorter. You are not required to pay back the loan advances or interest until the term of the loan is finished. In most reverse mortgages, no repayment is due until you die, sell your home, or permanently move away.

As with any big financial decisions, reverse mortgages carry some risks. Before you can apply for a reverse mortgage, you must meet with an independent third-party counseling service to ensure that this option is appropriate for you. For information about these counseling services, contact the National Home Equity Conversion Network (www.hud.gov or 800-569-4287) or the National Reverse Mortgage Lenders Association (www.reversemortgage.org or 202-939-1760). Also, to obtain a free copy of the reverse mortgage consumer guide *Home Made Money,* plus other helpful materials, contact AARP (www .aarp.org/revmort or 800-209-8085).[3]

Life Insurance Settlements

A creative way to pay long-term care expenses is through a financial arrangement known as a "life settlement," which is also sometimes called a "viatical settlement." This involves selling an existing life insurance policy to a third party—a person or an entity other than the company that issued the policy—for more than the policy's cash surrender value, but less than the net death benefit. In return, the policyholder receives tax-free proceeds, and the funds can be used for any purpose. Generally, individuals must have a life expectancy of five years or less in order to tap into this asset. Life settlements can be a valuable source of money, but they are not for everyone. They can have high transaction costs and tax consequences. And even if this idea is appealing, it can be hard to determine a fair price. It is important to consult with a trusted attorney, financial advisor, or insurance broker for advice on this option.

Rethinking the Living Situation

A question that inevitably arises for those tending to a person with AD is whether to consider moving him or her to another residence in light of the expected decline. The person with AD can conceivably remain in his or her own home indefinitely as long as informal and formal services are put in place as needed. As noted in Chapter 7, if the person with AD lives alone, several options need to be explored: enlisting the help of family and friends, hiring in-home help, moving into a relative's home, or relocating to a facility with supportive services. The option of living independently without some form of help is unrealistic. Furthermore, the level of help must gradually increase over time to correspond with growing impairments caused by the disease.

Many spouses of people with AD consider relocating to a smaller home or condominium for the sake of simplifying their lifestyle. Other spouses prefer to buy a larger home in anticipation of sharing it with a paid helper in the future. Still others consider moving into facilities that offer varying levels of care. Moving closer to family members and friends who may provide assistance may also be a good idea.

When considering the possibility of moving to a care facility, you do not need to think strictly in terms of licensed nursing homes, also known as intermediate-care or skilled-care facilities. These care facilities are not well suited for people in the early stages of AD and are intended mainly for individuals in later stages of the disease. In the United States, a growing trend is to create alternatives that afford greater autonomy and offer homier environments than traditional nursing homes. You need to be informed about these different options to choose the most appropriate living situation for your loved one with AD.

Retirement Communities

Most retirement communities were built originally with independent, healthy older individuals in mind. These communities have traditionally offered studio or one- or two-bedroom apartments, a common dining area and a meal plan, some housekeeping services, and a range of leisure activities. Fees are paid monthly, and entry fees are not required. It is expected that people living in retirement communities are fairly independent and will transition to a health-care facility only if needed. However, in recent years these facilities have seen a gradual shift toward accommodating residents of retirement communities with mild disabilities including the early stages of AD.

Although many retirement communities have added a separate health-care wing or facility, many do not have any additional levels of care. Most retirement communities have adapted to the needs of their residents by forming relationships with home-care agencies that provide additional services, ranging from a bath once a week to daily medication monitoring. These services are typically not included in the monthly fee and must be paid for privately, on a fee-for-service basis.

Assisted Living Facilities and Other Residential Care Facilities

Assisted living facilities (ALFs) refer to apartment-style living arrangements intended to serve those needing assistance with daily tasks by means of twenty-four-hour staff. ALFs have become increasingly popular in serving the needs of people with AD. The term *assisted living* has no standard definition, and many states do not require facilities to be licensed. Thus, there is a wide range of quality and services available in ALFs. They typically provide twenty-four-hour security, emergency call systems for each resident's apartment, two or three meals a day, housekeeping, laundry, transportation, medication management, recreational activities, and assistance with bathing, dressing, and toileting.

The cost and scope of services in ALFs range widely from place to place. Some facilities offer private apartments, while others offer just a private or shared room and bath. Many of these care facilities cater specifically to the needs of people with AD, who now compose the majority of people living in ALFs today. For the most part, the cost of living in an ALF is paid privately or with the aid of long-term care insurance, with costs running from $4,000 to $8,000 monthly. Most ALFs today are proprietary and are either privately owned or public businesses, with many of them belonging to large national chains.

Assisted living is really an umbrella term for many different types of housing options: board-and-care homes, residential facilities, and supportive housing. In some states, government agencies regulate and help pay for care provided in these facilities, while most states have chosen not to regulate or provide any form of payment. Either public health agencies or state departments of aging or social services can provide information about funding, laws, and policies governing each type of facility in your area. Another good source of information is the provider organization Assisted Living Federation of America (www .alfa.org).

Continuing Care Retirement Communities

Continuing care retirement communities (CCRCs) offer at least three levels of care: independent/retirement living, assisted living, and nursing home care. CCRCs are usually situated on campuses with several sections or buildings that accommodate hundreds of people. The basic premise is that older people in reasonably good health may want to first enjoy independent living in the retirement section but want the security of additional care, should it become necessary, in adjacent sections of the same community. Most CCRCs require a one-time entrance fee and then monthly payments thereafter. These fees vary by community, depending on the type of housing and services they offer. Other CCRCs operate on a rental basis, in which you would make monthly payments, but would not have to pay an entrance fee. Some CCRCs accept Medicaid reimbursement for nursing home care when residents deplete their assets, while most others rely on private payments or endowments.

The retirement and assisted living sections of CCRCs may be appropriate for people in the early stages of AD, while those in the later stages may need services available in the nursing home section. Married couples in which one spouse has AD may be well served in the retirement section for a long time into the disease, as long as the well spouse can manage day-to-day care, with or without extra services. Although the retirement section offers minimal services, additional services such as personal care can usually be purchased on a fee-for-service basis with an outside agency. Some communities require that all residents be relatively independent at the time of admission, while most others accept people with different levels of need. Admission requirements and costs vary from place to place. Some CCRCs are nonprofit, religiously affiliated facilities that belong to a provider organization known as Leading Age (www.leadingage.org), while others are proprietary and privately owned.

The array of possible living arrangements can seem confusing at first. If you are considering several care facilities, become a well-informed consumer. Shop around for the best fit in terms of services, costs, and location. The pros and cons of home-care options and residential-care facilities must be carefully weighed in light of the financial, social, and psychological resources of all concerned parties. The preferences of the person with AD should not be the sole priority. Rather, your needs as well as the concerns of others must be included in your decision-making process. In the final analysis, you must serve as the judge in determining if a move is worthwhile. This requires good communication with others who may be affected by the decision, so that their roles are clarified. For example, if a spouse expresses a desire to move because the new locale includes relatives who will help, then these expectations need to be shared with everyone. Likewise, if assisted living seems the best option to you, others need to know your rationale if you expect them to participate in ongoing care.

As a rule, relocation should happen sooner rather than later in the disease. People with AD are much more likely to make a positive adjustment to a new environment in the early stage of the disease than they are in later stages. Nevertheless, even for people in the early stage, a temporary worsening in memory, mood, and behavior is likely to occur when they move. Keeping up the daily routine of the person with AD and retaining favorite home furnishings and keepsakes may help to ease the transition. If you or someone else can be available for a short time to assist the person with AD in navigating the new surroundings, the adjustment process will be eased. Within a matter of weeks, the new home usually begins to feel familiar and the unpleasant effects of the move fade away. To help prepare you for a move and ease the transition, I recommend reading the short book, *Moving a Relative with Memory Loss: A Family Caregiver's Guide,* by Laurie White and Beth Spencer.[4]

Finding the Right Professionals

At every stage of the disease, you will need the expertise and support of competent and compassionate health-care professionals. Every person with AD should have one primary-care physician to coordinate care. Finding a physician who is experienced with AD and understands its impact on families must be your top priority. Physicians of internal medicine or family practice are typically involved in primary care and are often experienced in diagnosing and treating symptoms of AD as well as in addressing other medical problems that may arise. Finding a physician with specialty training and certification in geriatrics is ideal, but the number of board-certified "geriatricians" is relatively small at present.

Neurologists and neuropsychologists are best suited to diagnose AD and related brain disorders. Psychiatrists, psychologists, nurses, and social workers may be useful in assessing and treating the behavioral changes sometimes associated with the disease. To find a good physician or another health-care professional, inquire at a nearby hospital, clinic, adult day center, home-care agency, and the local chapter of the Alzheimer's Association. If the names of certain professionals are repeatedly suggested by your sources of information, then it is worth following these leads.

Fortunately, there are growing numbers of health-care professionals who are sensitive to the needs of those with AD and their families. First, they recognize that families are the main providers of care and deserve to be involved in all care decisions. These professionals realize that their role is limited mainly to providing consultation to families and supporting you in your key role in the life of the person with AD. This shared approach to care is not only realistic but quite helpful as well. Second, they make a point of communicating with families by listening to their needs and teaching them about the disease. They take the time to explain various treatment options as well as options not to treat. These sensitive professionals enable families to participate in decisions affecting the care of the person with AD and pay special attention to the opinions of the person most responsible for day-to-day care.

Good health care is no longer taken for granted by a consumer-oriented public. The rise in medical malpractice suits and complaints about managed-care organizations attest to the public's dissatisfaction with shoddy service. It is vitally important to find a health-care professional in whom you have confidence and who can be trusted over the long haul. You may need to shop around before you find the right professional or team of professionals. Choosing the right people to work with you will have lasting benefits.

Thus far, this book has addressed the major goals of making legal and financial plans, settling the living situation, and finding the right health-care professionals. Once you achieve these short-term goals, you can turn your attention to the ongoing goal of keeping the person with AD involved in meaningful activities. Again, achieving this goal cannot be met by you alone, so enlisting the help of others is vital to the well-being of both the person with AD and you. In the next chapter, I explain ways to engage people with AD in a variety of meaningful activities.

10 Keeping a Person with Alzheimer's Disease Active

To affect the quality of the day, that is the highest of arts.
Henry David Thoreau

Staying active is an essential part of a good quality of life for someone with AD. However, many activities that he or she formerly carried out with ease may no longer be feasible given the impairments in memory, thinking, and language caused by the disease. Therefore, you will need to structure and modify activities that promote well-being. And you will also need to take into account his or her abilities and disabilities when planning new activities. What is an activity? It's the stuff of everyday life. It can be something simple like making a sandwich or something complex like taking a trip to a foreign country. Activities may span the six dimensions of well-being (discussed previously on pages 74–75):

- emotional—opportunities to express feelings and release stress
- intellectual—opportunities to solve problems and make decisions
- physical—opportunities to participate in self-care, household tasks, exercise, sports, and recreation
- social—opportunities to be with people or pets
- spiritual—opportunities to connect with the divine with others or alone
- vocational—opportunities to use life skills and expertise

Far too many people with AD suffer from loneliness, helplessness, and boredom. As noted in Chapter 5, the antidotes to these problems include intimacy, community, and meaningful activities. Accommodating these human needs may require some work on your part. Since the person with AD cannot be expected to meet these needs alone, you and others must act to create opportunities. When you and others participate in activities with the person with AD, you allow him or her to use retained abilities, minimize deficits, preserve self-esteem, and enjoy closeness with others. Shared activities serve as reminders that life is worth living.

You may intuitively know the value of structured activities in your life, but the person with AD may no longer be capable of organizing and following routines without some aid. For example, daily meals provide a certain rhythm to life, but people with AD may become disoriented about time and forget to eat regularly. Planned mealtimes help them structure their time and provide a sense of daily order. Many people with AD worry about failing at certain tasks and may lose the initiative to try anything, be it routine or new and different, unless encouraged to do so. Fear and embarrassment may isolate them from others, but when provided with appropriate activities, they will feel successful and connected to their surroundings. For example, with daily activities such as meals, you can ask the person with AD to help out, even in a small way. The right kind of activity can also help family members and friends enjoy doing something *with* the person with AD instead of *for* that individual. Such activities enable the person with AD to interact with others and allow you to enlist others' help. The key is to select enjoyable activities to keep momentum going. Instead of doing something different every day, the person with AD may thrive on routine and repetitive activities as long as they are meaningful and enjoyable. A schedule of activities or calendar of events may serve as a useful reminder and create a rhythm that you and the person with AD find useful.

Involving Others

It is important to involve others in planning, initiating, and executing informal and formal activities. You will eventually need help and enlisting the help of others in doing things is a good way to start.

Moreover, it is unrealistic and psychologically unhealthy for you to be responsible for organizing all activities at all times. You may feel that joint activities that are mutually satisfying require little or no effort on your part. However, both you and the person with AD need time apart for the sake of personal renewal, so engaging in separate activities from time to time is important. To successfully enlist the help of other family members and friends, a few steps should be taken.

First, it is safe to assume that many people do not know what to say or do in relation to someone with AD. It is natural for others either to pretend that nothing is wrong or to stereotype the person as completely helpless. You will need to honestly address both of these extremes with an explanation of the facts about the disease in order to dispel myths and answer questions. Your insight and encouragement can help friends and relatives adapt to disease-related changes and to be of greater service to both you and the person with AD. They may need information about how to communicate effectively with the diagnosed person. Or they may need to learn how to maximize her or his remaining abilities. You can use educational brochures, books, and videos to reinforce your explanations.

Second, keep in mind that other people do not have the kind of contact with the person with AD that enables you to understand the nuances of the disease. Simply telling them about the disease or getting them to read an educational pamphlet is not enough; give them opportunities to have firsthand experiences. Encourage them to spend time alone with the person with AD, perhaps for a few hours or even a few days. It is always eye opening! There is no quicker way for you to gain an ally than by letting someone get this direct experience.

Sometimes other people may casually offer to help you or the person with AD. You should take such offers seriously and be prepared with an idea or two in order to engage them as soon as possible. Others often need you to give them ideas about how to be of assistance. It is important to be specific and concrete with your instructions. For example, you may want to see a play at a local theater and feel uncomfortable taking the person with AD with you. Asking someone else to be a companion for the person with AD in your absence is a good way of introducing other people to the helping role. You should be prepared to suggest some activities that can be done while you are away, such as making a snack, watching a favorite movie, playing a game, or looking through a scrapbook together.

Just as you adapted to the changes brought on by the disease and altered your expectations of the person with AD, so must other family members and friends. In the long haul, loyal family members and friends may prove indispensable in sharing the care. I have heard many experienced family members express regret that they did not call on others for help until they found themselves in dire need. It cannot be said enough: Do not hesitate to ask for help!

People who care for loved ones with AD often say, "You find out who are your true friends in the course of this disease." Sometimes those you expected to help, especially those who live nearby, may be unavailable. They may have other priorities or lack the emotional capacity to spend time with a relative or friend who has AD. You may feel disappointed or resentful when this happens, but if others do not respond to a direct approach, it is best not to press further. Precious time and energy may be wasted on futile efforts and further disappointment. Nevertheless, keep the channels of communication open, since these relatives and friends may eventually come around in their own time and way.

Try to maintain nurturing relationships or develop new contacts. You and the person with AD need people who can provide practical help and moral support. These may include friends, siblings, in-laws, neighbors, children, grandchildren, and even great-grandchildren. If such helpers are not readily available, finding other people who are in similar circumstances may be a good alternative. For example, teaming up with other spouses or adult children responsible for relatives with AD, through support groups or formal activity programs, may be useful.

Dealing with Depression

As noted in Chapter 1, lack of initiative or apathy sometimes accompanies AD. As a general rule, it is not a good idea to force an apathetic person to take part in an activity, even though it may be beneficial. However, gentle persuasion may motivate someone to participate and enjoy meaningful activities. Related to apathy is the more troubling problem of depression that co-exists with AD in up to half of cases. Depression is generally under-diagnosed and not well treated.

In addition to apathy, according to the National Institute of Mental Health, symptoms of depression may include:

- difficulty concentrating, remembering details, and making decisions
- feelings of guilt, worthlessness, and/or helplessness
- feelings of hopelessness and/or pessimism
- insomnia, early-morning wakefulness, or excessive sleeping
- irritability, restlessness
- loss of interest in activities or hobbies once pleasurable, including sex
- overeating or appetite loss
- persistent aches or pains, headaches, cramps, or digestive problems that do not ease even with treatment
- persistent sad, anxious, or "empty" feelings
- thoughts of suicide, suicide attempts

There are at least two interrelated causes of depression: psychological disturbance and biological changes. Depression is a normal psychological reaction to loss. For people with AD, the gradual losses of many intellectual abilities can result in feelings of depression. Depression may also be caused by chemical changes in the brain. It is well known that people with AD have reduced levels of many brain chemicals, including serotonin, which is associated with depression. Regardless of the underlying cause, every effort should be made to diagnose and alleviate symptoms of depression.

Antidepressants and psychological therapies are the main treatments for depression. The class of drugs most commonly used for treatment today are known as SSRIs (selective serotonin reuptake inhibitors), and they essentially boost the level of serotonin in the brain. SSRIs include brand names like Zoloft, Lexapro, Paxil, Prozac, and Celexa. Because responses to drugs vary from person to person, different drugs and different dosages may have to be tried before improvement is seen, but it is usually expected within two weeks.

In addition to an antidepressant, someone with AD who is depressed may benefit from psychological therapies for the sake of talking about one's feelings with a mental health professional. Controversy exists over the value of this type of treatment. Since AD impairs one's capacity to create and retain new memories, carrying over ideas and insights from one talk therapy session to the next is obviously problematic. Nevertheless, some people with AD may benefit from talking with a professional about their feelings of depression. Other things that may help are increasing the amount of time spent doing activities that the person enjoys and engaging in various forms of physical exercise.

Selecting Appropriate Activities

Although people with AD in the early stages may have the energy to participate in activities, they often lack the ability to get going or to sequence the steps properly—much like having a car's motor running with the gears stuck in neutral. Without assistance, many people with the disease become confused about how to proceed with even the simplest task. One woman talked about wanting the help of others: "People can help bring me out. With this disease, you can get lost inside yourself." People with AD tend to withdraw from activities such as household tasks, social events, and hobbies if they are not regularly encouraged to continue them. Therefore, your first priority is to select activities that are geared to the individual's needs, abilities, and preferences.

Many people with AD initially resist invitations to participate in activities and need some encouragement. You can set the right tone by narrowing or eliminating the number of available options. For example, it is preferable to offer two choices such as, "Would you like to take a walk around the block or take a walk to the park?" instead of asking, "Would you like to take a walk?" Without options, the second question leaves room for an easy refusal. You may also be assertive in suggesting, "Let's go for a walk," or you may insist, "We need to take a walk right now." In either case, the person with AD is unlikely to refuse. Once he or she is involved in an activity, any inertia or resistance may vanish.

A continual process of adaptation is needed to keep up with the changes and needs of the person with AD. If the person is no longer able to plan, initiate, or complete activities independently, you will need to determine which steps are still possible with some help. For example, a hobby such as painting may require step-by-step direction from you or someone else. Pastimes requiring a great deal of concentration, such as playing cards, needlepoint or reading, may prove too taxing. As a result, you may want to introduce other activities such as taking a walk, listening to music, singing songs, or watching a movie. Again, expect a process of trial and error to learn what works.

When selecting the proper activities for the person with AD, keep her or his personal preferences in mind. For example, some people do not like to be served but are quite willing and able to serve others. Some people are content to be passive observers while others insist on being active participants. Although such preferences may change over time in some cases, they generally remain the same well into the disease process. People who have always enjoyed reading may continue to do so despite their inability to recall what they have read. As the disease worsens, however, their desire for a variety and complexity of activities diminishes. Simple, familiar, and predictable activities may become more satisfying than a busy lifestyle. Recognizing and adapting to such changing needs and preferences requires your continued flexibility.

You also need to adjust each activity to meet individualized needs, such as whether the person with AD can participate independently or as a passive observer. In her book about activities for people with AD, *Doing Things: A Guide to Programming Activities for Persons with Alzheimer's Disease and Related Disorders,* occupational therapist Jitka Zgola explains the concept of "activity grading" that allows someone to participate in the same activity at different levels of needs and abilities.[1] In the example below, the steps involved in baking cookies are broken down to illustrate how one can participate in this activity at different levels. At the highest level of involvement, the person with AD would be capable of executing all the steps to make cookies, from start to finish. At the lowest level of involvement, the person with AD would passively observe someone else carry out the many steps. This concept can be applied to virtually any type of activity.

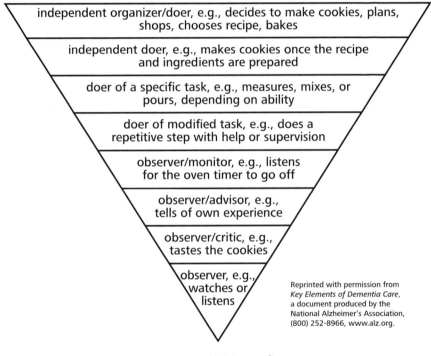

independent organizer/doer, e.g., decides to make cookies, plans, shops, chooses recipe, bakes

independent doer, e.g., makes cookies once the recipe and ingredients are prepared

doer of a specific task, e.g., measures, mixes, or pours, depending on ability

doer of modified task, e.g., does a repetitive step with help or supervision

observer/monitor, e.g., listens for the oven timer to go off

observer/advisor, e.g., tells of own experience

observer/critic, e.g., tastes the cookies

observer, e.g., watches or listens

Reprinted with permission from *Key Elements of Dementia Care*, a document produced by the National Alzheimer's Association, (800) 252-8966, www.alz.org.

FIGURE 10.1 Activity grading

The Importance of Everyday Activities

When choosing activities that best fit the abilities, limitations, and preferences of the person with AD, it is important to begin with activities that "normalize" her or his life. In other words, choose activities that are consistent with his or her past and fit into a daily routine. If the person is used to watching sports on television or listening to music, there is no need to change habits. If taking a walk in the neighborhood is part of the daily routine, then it should continue. Similarly, you can encourage the person with AD to help with things such as cutting up vegetables, folding laundry, or raking leaves. In this sense, almost everything can be considered an activity in which the person with AD can be engaged, at least to some degree. In her memoir about caring for her father with AD, *Measure of the Heart: A Father's Alzheimer's, a Daughter's Return,* Mary Ellen Geist recounts his fascination with using a vacuum:

> He seemed to have a knack for it. He could not remember how to turn the machine on or off, but once the sound of the vacuum kicked in, he suddenly remembered and began expertly cleaning the carpet and floors. Sometimes, even when the house was clean, Mom would have him vacuum so he'd feel useful and she'd get a break.[2]

It is often a good idea to simplify familiar activities. For example, if the person with AD is accustomed to doing the laundry from beginning to end, then just folding the clothes when they're dry may be rewarding enough. As long as people with AD feel part of an activity, it makes no difference whether they participate in every step. Personal satisfaction, the highest possible degree of involvement, and the chance to do something enjoyable together count more than the end result. The process is what matters most of all. One woman whose husband has AD learned this lesson the hard way:

> I used to get upset with Lou for taking so long to get dressed in the morning. I jumped in to help him a couple of times, and he snapped at me for treating him like a child. I had to realize that it was in his best interest to let him do it by himself, no matter how long it took. He felt good about it, and that, in itself, was pleasing to me.

If the person with AD finds an activity enjoyable, there is no reason why it should not be done over and over again. In fact, repeating the same activity may allow for more opportunities to feel successful.

Many activities that the person considered simple or boring in the past may now seem satisfying. For example, one man discovered that his wife with AD enjoyed taking long drives in their car and was not concerned about a destination. In another case, a woman was surprised to discover that her husband with AD liked cutting out coupons from magazines and newspapers. A daughter was flabbergasted that her mother had a newfound interest in watching golf on television.

Activities that might be perceived as childish or demeaning, such as using crayons and coloring books, should be avoided, although the person with AD must be allowed to define the personal meaning of a particular activity. New and different interests may develop. For example, to the surprise of everyone, one woman with AD began collecting baseball cards, and her collection became a focus of activity among her circle of family and friends. In another case, a man with AD enjoyed reading storybooks to his young grandchildren and playing the board game Chutes and Ladders with them.

Intellectual Activities

There is some debate about the value of stimulating the person with AD through intellectual activities such as memory exercises, games, and puzzles. As already noted, there is no solid evidence that intellectual activities help to improve the brain's function or slow the progression of the disease. Furthermore, the person with AD may feel frustrated by her or his inability to perform these activities. Again, the chief aim of such activities should be to enable the person to use remaining abilities instead of trying to improve memory. If such activities are still enjoyable for someone with the disease, then he or she should continue until they are no longer enjoyable. For example, many people with AD enjoy reading magazines and newspapers, although they may recall little or nothing of what they have read. The same might be said for those of us without memory loss, but that does not keep us from reading for the pure sake of enjoyment. If someone with AD enjoys taxing his or her mental abilities, then why not honor those efforts?

At all times, a person with AD should be given opportunities to use his or her remaining abilities to the extent possible without crossing the line to frustration. Pressuring someone with AD to "exercise" the brain through memorizing word lists or concentrating harder on a task is not helpful. In fact, efforts intended to have someone with AD "learn" or "remember" may evoke or intensify feelings of inadequacy. Being able to maximize someone's remaining abilities with minimal risk of failure, however, can help to enhance self-esteem and autonomy. People with AD may still derive enjoyment from games and puzzles if they enjoyed these activities in the past, but simplifying and adapting these activities may be necessary. Board games such as Scrabble and Trivial Pursuit or television game shows such as *Wheel of Fortune* and *Jeopardy* may be suitable and can be enjoyed by adults and children alike. Crossword and jigsaw puzzles can be done with other people or alone. Participating in games such as board games, dice, and blocks with young children may serve two purposes: bringing the generations together and teaching children how to have fun with the person who has AD.

Card games typically require a good grasp of rules as well as a working memory, and therefore may not be a good choice. However, some people with AD retain an uncanny degree of skill in these games and should continue playing them as long as they enjoy them. For example, one woman who had been a bridge player for more than fifty years was able to participate actively in her bridge club long after she was diagnosed with AD. Again, sometimes the activity may need to be modified. When one man with AD no longer wished to play pinochle, he agreed to partner with his wife in playing the game with their friends. Through this simple accommodation, the whole group remained intact.

Traveling

People in the early stages of AD may continue to travel and take vacations if precautions are taken to minimize potential problems. In the later stages, they may feel too disoriented and anxious when they are away from home to enjoy travel. Since you may have a window of opportunity for traveling right now, plan to act soon if you or your loved one with the disease desire to travel or take a vacation, or you may regret it later.

Generally, the person with AD should not travel alone except under controlled conditions. For instance, flying from one airport to another may be feasible when someone is available to help at the beginning and end of the trip. However, even the best-laid plans can go awry, so each situation should be carefully assessed. It is always best for the person with the disease to have a traveling companion for the sake of safety and enjoyment. The Transportation Security Administration (TSA) has a toll-free help line number, (855) 787-2227, to provide information for passengers with disabilities and their families before they fly and to ease passage through security checkpoints.

People with AD may tire easily in unfamiliar surroundings, so a slower-than-average pace or regular rest periods may be needed while away from home. Travel usually disrupts the daily routine, which can trigger confusion in someone with AD who does fine at home. Maintaining routines as much as possible while traveling may reduce this risk. Having additional traveling companions, to share the responsibilities as well as the fun of travel, may make a trip more enjoyable for everyone.

As long as you closely monitor the whereabouts of the person with AD during a trip, he or she has little chance of getting lost. Just in case, though, the person with the disease should always wear some form of identification. ID bracelets and necklaces inscribed with a toll-free phone number for a computerized registry are available through the "Medic Alert + Safe Return Program" of the Alzheimer's Association; check with your local chapter for details. A recent photo of the person should also be kept on hand to aid local law-enforcement agencies in a search. And thanks to global positioning system (GPS) technology, it is possible to track someone with AD who may have become lost or wandered away. Many such helpful location-tracking products are available today, including the Alzheimer's Association's Comfort Zone Check-In. One of the most fascinating innovations is GPS shoes, which will notify you if the wearer has walked outside a predetermined area.

Participating in Social Events

The person with AD may also still enjoy social events if proper precautions are taken. Overwhelming sights, sounds, and numbers of people may prove confusing and lead the person to withdraw, so limit how much they're exposed to potential sources of confusion. For example, instead of a several-hour event, something shorter may be enough. On special occasions such as holiday gatherings, weddings, and birthday parties, the person with AD may feel alone in a crowd unless others are willing to engage him or her one-on-one. Several people may share this responsibility, taking turns to make sure that he or she has an enjoyable time. Sensitizing others to the likes and dislikes of the person with AD in advance of these occasions should be part of planning for a specific event.

Even gatherings with a few people may prove too taxing if conditions are unfavorable. For example, the rules of golf may no longer be easy to remember, causing embarrassment to the person with AD if they play a game. Forgetting the names of others in a small group may also be a source of frustration. A receptive attitude on the part of others, coupled with a willingness to modify group activities to suit the person with AD, will make socialization easier for everyone concerned. Again, this requires that others be made aware of the person's needs and be given suggestions about minimizing confusion (for example, not asking questions about recent events).

Reminiscing

Although AD inhibits people from creating new memories, memories of the distant past are usually well preserved in the early stages. Therefore, reminiscing may be a truly enjoyable activity for someone with the disease. While hearing the same stories over and over may grow tiresome for the listener, this may be an ideal time for you to gather information about family history. One way to do this is through video interviews. The person with AD can begin by telling his or her life story with some direction by an interviewer. There are several interview guides available to facilitate sharing of one's personal story. Such conversations provide a permanent record that can later be reviewed and appreciated by others. Edited versions of these interviews make beautiful gifts and lasting reminders of a family's history.

Scrapbooks, photographs, and other keepsakes may trigger conversations about personal background and historical events. Discussions about the past may also offer valuable insights to younger people and help link generations. Details about one's heritage are often lost with the death of older members of the family who have not told or been asked about their family history. Reminiscing is a valuable way of ensuring that does not happen.

You can also help the person with AD tap into past memories by visiting important places, listening to favorite music, watching old movies, and reviewing photo albums. You might transfer old 8mm films to a DVD for easy viewing. Even handling a set of tools or cooking utensils can bring forth old stories. By creatively stimulating all the senses—sight, sound, touch, smell, and taste—you can help evoke countless old memories. For example, one woman with AD spent two hours daily at a local garden recalling her wealth of knowledge about plants, trees, and flowers.

Spiritual and Religious Practices

Traditional religious practices can also trigger long-term or distant memory. Many people are members of the same religious organization throughout their lifetime, and numerous aspects of religious practice, such as familiar prayers, rituals, and hymns, may be firmly preserved in memory and may be recalled for personal and group worship. Catholics, for example, may remember how to use their rosaries to repeat the series of memorized prayers.

The structured and predictable order of worship used in churches, synagogues, and mosques may be comfortingly familiar to a person with AD who has trouble handling spontaneous situations. Participating in religious activities should be encouraged if they are part of the person's heritage. If possible, the members of the religious congregation, especially the leaders, should be educated and sensitized to the needs of people with AD. Learning about AD can go a long way toward helping stay connected with members who are coping with the disease. On this topic, I recommend the booklet, *You Are One of Us: Successful Clergy/Church Connections to Alzheimer's Families* by Lisa Gwyther.[3]

Music, too, can evoke many old memories, especially in religious settings, and a person with AD may recall lyrics and melodies of songs with little or no prompting. In fact, as the ability to communicate through words diminishes, the power of music to evoke thoughts and feelings should not be underestimated. In his personal account of living with AD, Cary Henderson makes several references to his renewed appreciation for music and the "consoling" nature of symphonic music. Of course, musical tastes vary, and no single type of music is pleasing to all people with AD. Knowing about the person's past preferences may be useful in choosing the type of music that may be appealing now, but preferences may change. In *My Journey into Alzheimer's Disease,* clergyman Robert Davis describes his irritation with certain religious music that he used to enjoy. One man I know discovered that his wife with AD had a renewed appreciation for big-band music, so he put together a collection of her favorites that she listened to every day. An iPod or a similar electronic device is an easy way to enjoy musical selections without any distractions.

Helping the Person with AD Maintain Physical Health

Primary ways of helping people with AD maintain their physical health include ensuring that they get a proper diet and regular exercise. Again, people with AD usually cannot handle these priorities alone and need assistance. Regarding diet, AD itself has no restrictions, special foods or supplements indicated. However, coexisting medical problems such as heart disease, hypertension, or diabetes usually necessitate certain diets, and people with AD need help to maintain those diets. You or someone else also needs to ensure that your loved one is eating balanced meals. He or she should be encouraged to participate in any number of food-related steps from making a grocery list to shopping, preparing the meal, and washing dishes. It should be noted that sometimes people with the disease crave sweets and lose interest in nutritious foods. This craving may be related to changes in their sense of taste caused by the disease. This craving should not be discouraged as long as other foods are being consumed. Cigarette smoking and alcohol should also be curbed for safety reasons or should be closely supervised. It is surprising that people with AD often forget about using cigarettes and alcohol when these things are no longer available.

Exercise is another vital part of maintaining good physical health. Muscle strength, joint flexibility, balance, bone density, and cardiopulmonary outputs are threatened by lack of physical exertion. Regular exercise can help the body maintain, repair, and improve itself. Exercise promotes good sleep patterns as well as emotional well-being. People with AD can carry out a variety of physical activities in the course of a normal day. Walking is an easy form of exercise that should be done daily. No set amount of time or distance is prescribed for walking, but each outing should offer a mix of exertion and enjoyment. If the person with AD can no longer drive, then walking or bicycling to nearby destinations are good alternatives if disorientation is not an issue. Stretching the neck, arms, shoulders, waist, hips, legs, and knees can be done with or without a structured routine. Exercise equipment such as a stationary bikes or treadmills are also easy to use with proper supervision. It is always wise to check with the person's physician and a fitness instructor in case an individualized exercise program is needed. Without even having to leave the house, the person with AD can get exercise by doing daily chores such as housekeeping and yard work.

Structured exercise classes are available through community centers and other recreational programs. Working out at a health club probably requires someone to help negotiate the surroundings. One woman with AD stuck to her routine of participating three times weekly in an exercise program at a local swimming pool, thanks to the cooperation of her swimming group. A man with AD worked out regularly at a gym under the guidance of a personal trainer. Numerous workout videos and manuals are also available in modified formats for older people. Organized games that rely on motor skills, such as bowling, shuffleboard, and croquet, may also be therapeutic. People with AD can enjoy other indoor and outdoor activities like swimming and golf if modifications are made, such as relaxing the scoring rules in a golf game. Experimenting with different physical activities before they become a part of the person's daily life is always a good idea.

Support Groups

Support groups for people in the early stages of AD exist in most major urban areas, usually under the auspices of the Alzheimer's Association or big medical centers. Support groups are typically led by professionals and offer a supportive atmosphere to achieve several goals. Typically support groups include eight to twelve people with AD, who meet to discuss common concerns and enjoy mutual support. These group meetings are useful for gaining knowledge about the disease and exchanging coping strategies.

Most support groups meet weekly for a period of eight to ten weeks, but some meet monthly on an ongoing basis. While the people with AD are meeting, their family members and friends usually participate in professionally led groups in an adjacent room to discuss their own agendas. Both groups often then come together for a time of socialization. Members of these support groups tend to bond quickly and derive much satisfaction from their participation, and some people choose to see one another on a social basis, too. For example, a support group organized by the House of Welcome in Northfield, Illinois, spawned a monthly "Supper Club" for couples in which one partner has AD. Such gatherings are natural in light of common interests and needs. Problems like forgetting names and losing track of conversations trigger no embarrassment in a peer group. The research conducted thus far shows that these groups offer many benefits to people with AD and their care partners. Taking part in supports groups may be useful in reducing social isolation, enhancing self-esteem, and coping better with memory loss. One woman noted her husband's positive response to participation in a support group: "He used to hide his problems, and now he is much more open in letting others know what he needs. I think the group gave him the confidence that having Alzheimer's disease is no cause for shame."

Members of a group in Prince George, British Columbia, offered the following comments about the benefits of their participation:

> When I was first diagnosed, it was quite a shock. But then I came and met these interesting people. It means a lot to know you are not alone.

> I am very thankful the group was suggested by my doctor. To meet these people experienced with this condition has been so supportive and so much fun. When you're diagnosed, you feel so alone—and then you come here, and it feels like a family.

> You don't have to be on guard here; just be as we are. We exchange ideas and laugh.

Though support groups are not for everyone, they can provide a wonderful outlet for some people with AD. Often people with AD need prompting to try out these groups, but they are usually quick to adapt to these enjoyable and meaningful gatherings. Likewise, family members and friends are usually grateful for the knowledge gained and support received in early-stage support groups.

To find out about a support group in your area, contact the local chapter of the Alzheimer's Association (www.alz.org or 800-272-3900) or the Alzheimer Society (www.alzheimer.ca or 416-488-8772). If a group does not exist in your area, you might encourage one of these organizations to start one.

Activity Programs

A small but growing number of activity-focused programs for persons in the early stages of AD have also been established in recent years. These programs are usually sponsored by an adult day center where the majority of participants have AD but at later stages. Although participants in these early-stage programs have opportunities to talk about their thoughts and feelings about living with AD, their contact mainly revolves around specific activities or events. For example, a group may take on a community gardening project, sort canned goods at a local food bank, or stuff envelopes for mailings. These projects can instill pride and self-worth. Like any enjoyable activity, however, the goal is not to produce concrete results as much as it is to enable group members to enjoy working with others. For example, at the St. Ann Center for Intergenerational Care in Milwaukee, daily activities with children offer immeasurable joy, especially to many older women with AD who spent their younger years caring for their own children.

A recreational group or a formal outing is primarily aimed at having fun, but other benefits usually accrue as well. These activities are typically led by professionals who provide organization and structure designed for the needs and preferences of people with AD. Numerous organizations have begun early-stage activity programs in recent years, and each program seems to have its own unique style and agenda. On-site activities, such as intellectual games, physical exercise, and discussions about music, art, and history, as well as field trips such as restaurant lunches and picnics, are common activities. Here are a few fine examples:

- CJE Senior Life, based in Chicago, sponsors a "Culture Bus" that allows people in the early stages of AD to take part in guided tours of cultural attractions and enjoy lunch together in ten weekly sessions.

- The University of Michigan sponsors several weekly activity programs for people in the early stages of AD and mild cognitive impairment at its Silver Club adult day center in Ann Arbor, Michigan.

- The twice weekly "Mind Matters" program sponsored by the North Shore Senior Center in Northfield, Illinois, offers a range of activities for people with early-stage AD and mild cognitive impairment.

- The "Brain Fitness Club" meets twice weekly at the First United Methodist Church in Winter Park, Florida, to enable people with AD to exercise their minds and bodies under the direction of professionals and college students.

- The weekly "Expressions" program sponsored by Advocate Lutheran Adult Day Services in Des Plaines, Illinois, offers a variety of intellectual, physical, and social activities for people in the early stages of AD.

- The weekly "Mind in Motion" program sponsored by the Alzheimer's Society of British Columbia is held at numerous sites and offers 45 minutes of physical exercise led by a fitness instructor followed by 60 minutes of social activities for people in the early stages of AD and their care partners.

To find out about an activity program in your area, contact an adult day center through the National Adult Day Services Association at www.nadsa.org or (877) 745-1440.

Since 2006 New York's Museum of Modern Art (MOMA) has sponsored monthly programs for people with AD and their care partners during non-public hours in which art galleries and special exhibits are viewed and discussed with staff and volunteers. Not only is this "Meet Me at MOMA" program popular, but research has shown the many social and emotional benefits for participants. This successful program has now been replicated at dozens of museums across the United States and Canada. Again, if such a program does not exist in your local area, encourage a museum director to get in touch with MOMA's department of education at www.moma.org/meetme or (212) 408-6347.

MOMA's program highlights the value of viewing and discussing art but engaging people with AD in other creative arts is often beneficial too. Painting, drawing, photography, writing, story telling, dance, poetry, and music can be done alone or in groups. Many of these activities take place at senior centers or park and recreation centers. Also, art therapists and music therapists can be hired to provide one-on-one sessions that can yield remarkable results.

Pets and Plants

Most people have had pets at some point in their life. Caring for animals can be a big responsibility as well as a source of enjoyment. People with AD may be quite capable of sharing the work of caring for pets and also may derive a sense of purpose from this responsibility. They may be delighted to have a relationship with a creature that offers unconditional love. One woman with AD noted, "I had so many responsibilities being taken away from me that getting a dog proved to be the one thing that I could still handle well. And my dog expects nothing out of me!" A man with AD reported that his dog provided a good reason to exercise: "I have a dog that needs to be run every day. So we run about two miles together. The dog more or less drags me, but it's still fun. I have a regular route and see neighbors along the way."

As pet owners know, however, having an animal in your life entails certain responsibilities and considerations. Any animal requires training and upkeep, and this effort requires both time and energy. Allergic reactions to pets may be another consideration. Some living situations prohibit the presence of pets, although a growing number of residential care facilities allow residents to have dogs. But any "drawbacks" of pet ownership can be minimized. For example, dogs that have already been trained may be available through the local Humane Society. In the case of a puppy, he or she can be trained with the help of an obedience school. Such initial efforts may have long-lasting benefits. Other types of animals such as cats and birds might also be a better fit, as they require little or no training and are easier to maintain than dogs.

Plants are another option for engaging the person with AD. Growing houseplants or gardening is a relatively easy way of connecting with nature and involves a number of activities that can be done together or on a solo basis. Gardening also requires effort, but the size and scope of indoor and outdoor gardening can be scaled to meet the desired effect. One man who cares for his wife with AD reports that they happily spend several hours daily tending their large garden: "We have always enjoyed this hobby, so I figured we should keep it up as long as possible. We don't get as much done now as we did in the past, but it keeps us both busy." Outdoor tasks such as planting, fertilizing, watering, transplanting, and harvesting fruits and vegetables can be a year-round activity in some locales. Indoor gardening, ranging from maintaining a variety of plants to a full-blown greenhouse, can also be a focal point of daily activity.

* * * * * * * *

Providing meaningful activities to someone with AD requires time, energy, and creativity. It is an ongoing challenge, and one person cannot meet this challenge indefinitely. It is essential to involve others as soon as possible so that they may share in the important responsibility of enhancing the quality of life for the person with AD. At the same time, you must also learn to care for yourself. Since you are so vital to the well-being of the person with AD, a commitment to nurturing yourself will ultimately benefit everyone involved. This topic is the focus of the remaining three chapters.

PART III

Caring for Yourself

11 Self-Renewal for Family and Friends

When we truly care for ourselves, it becomes possible to care more profoundly about other people. The more alert and sensitive we are to our own needs, the more loving and generous we can be toward others.

Eda LeShan

So far, this book has focused for the most part on understanding and meeting the needs of the person with AD. However, the importance of maintaining your own well-being cannot be overstated. Caring for someone with the disease requires great demands on your time and energy. You may feel as if your life is being turned upside down because of your changing roles and responsibilities. You may feel tested in body, mind, and spirit in ways that you did not think imaginable. If proper steps are not taken to remain healthy on these interconnected levels, a host of problems may ensue. In fact, there is a strong chance that you will suffer bad consequences. The good news is that you can reduce this possibility and learn how to manage the many stressors associated with caring for someone with AD.

In light of the growing population of older adults in recent decades and the resulting growth in the number of people affected by AD, relatives and friends involved in their care have been studied extensively by hundreds of social researchers. These studies have described the complex challenges of caring for people with AD, including the potential outcomes on the well-being of those directly involved in care. What is clear from these studies is that caring for someone with AD is risky business. Numerous studies attest to the potential for physical and mental exhaustion. One survey showed that family members spend an average of one hundred hours a week providing supervision or some measure of care if they live with the person with the disease. Problems such as depression, anxiety, insomnia, social isolation, and various stress-related illnesses are far too common. Excessive use of alcohol or drugs as well as weight gain or weight loss are sure signs that something is awry. Virtually all of the research studies point out that these negative effects may be minimized or avoided through a variety of "self-care" practices.

Attitude Matters

Perhaps the most interesting and promising finding of research studies concerns the importance of attitude and perspective in determining how well one copes with the stressors of caring for someone with AD. People with a pessimistic outlook are prone to feel burdened and have other negative experiences, whereas such outcomes are less for people with a positive outlook. As a result, it has been shown that the severity of someone's AD symptoms is not a predictor of how well or how poorly someone responds to the stressors of caring for someone with the disease. For example, one spouse might be "falling apart" due to the other spouse's AD in the early stages, whereas another spouse might be coping rather well with a spouse who is in the advanced stages of the disease. Although you cannot control the progression of a person's disease, it is possible to choose your attitude in response to his or her symptoms. This approach can be summed up in the old age: "You cannot control the wind, but you can adjust your sails."

If you are the one primarily responsible for someone with AD, it is absolutely essential that you take care of yourself while caring for him or her—for both your sakes. Since your life and the life of the person with AD are intertwined, your physical, emotional, and spiritual well-being directly affects her or him. Renewing your personal energy on a regular basis enables you to meet your goal of providing good care. Conversely, the person with AD suffers if you are in poor shape. Keep in mind the following analogy. Prior to an airplane's departure, flight attendants routinely instruct passengers how to use an oxygen mask in the event of an emergency. This is an important message intended to save lives. Passengers are told to put on their own mask first. Only then are they supposed to help others around them or else they might not be capable of helping others. Likewise, your personal needs are just as important as the needs of the person with AD—perhaps more so.

Paying attention to and meeting your own needs is not selfish. One woman I know commented on the need to continue enjoying life in spite of her husband's disease: "The biggest misunderstanding about this disease is that as soon as you're diagnosed, you're dead. People don't realize that there is life beyond the diagnosis, and that's what I'm trying to prove. He can still have a good life and so can I." Similarly, a man I know described caring for his wife as "The Alzheimer's Project." He learned that he would neither outlive her nor give her optimal care unless he cared for himself, too. In Marilyn Mitchell's memoir about caring for her friend with AD she notes, "Without respite, single-handedly caring for someone is a perilous undertaking, and because this is so, caretakers must allow themselves to seek help."[1]

You can do many things to maintain your well-being. You will gradually discover what works best for you. Other care partners or your own circle of friends may offer friendly advice, but you must ultimately choose what is best for you in developing a regular plan of self-care.

Listening to Your Body and Mind

The body-mind connection is a two-way street. That is, you can improve your physical well-being by maintaining a positive outlook, but you can also improve your outlook by tending to your physical well-being. If you are feeling down, it is more important than ever to eat well, exercise regularly, enjoy recreational or social activities, and get plenty of rest. Routine medical and dental checkups should also be maintained. It is all too easy to overlook these basic matters as your focus shifts to the needs of the person with AD.

Proper nutrition is essential to maintaining your physical well-being and so eating regular and balanced meals should be part of your daily routine. Keep in mind, too, that the many of the tasks associated with meals can be enjoyed with the person with AD. Planning, purchasing, and preparing healthy foods should be a central focus of your daily life. The "My Plate" guidelines (see Figure 11.1 below) describe what to eat each day based on the dietary recommendations set by the U.S. Department of Agriculture (www.ChooseMyPlate.gov). My Plate calls for eating or drinking from five basic food groups to get the nutrients you need on a daily basis, and at the same time, the right amount of calories to maintain a good weight. The recommended amount from each food group depends on one's sex, age, and level of physical activity.

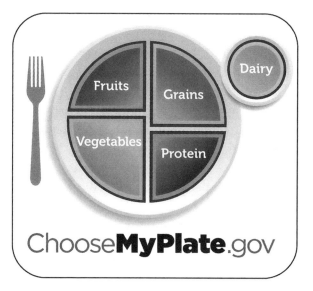

FIGURE 11.1 MyPlate (Source: U.S. Department of Agriculture)

A good daily diet generally consists of eating healthy foods from these five food groups:

1. fruits or 100 percent fruit juice
2. vegetables or 100 percent vegetable juice
3. grains (whole and refined)

4. protein food (such as meat, poultry, seafood, eggs, processed soy products, and nuts)

5. dairy (milk, milk-based products, and soymilk)

Cheese and ice cream contain both added sugars and fats. It is also vital that you incorporate exercise into your daily routine. Activities such as housekeeping and gardening are usually not strenuous enough to burn a lot of calories or to get your heart and lungs really working. Join a health club or try out yoga, weight training, jogging, or aerobics. If these don't appeal to you, then take a brisk walk for a mile or ride a stationary bike every day. You can play golf or swim alone or with others. But whether you choose a solo or group activity, the key is to be regularly physically active. One man whose wife has AD noted, "I try to do something for about an hour every day—mostly walking and bicycling but some canoeing and cross-country skiing when weather permits. I probably do more than necessary, but I feel pretty good. Doing something can start a cycle of feeling better, doing more, and feeling even better." One woman whose husband has the disease reported, "I attend a fitness center four mornings a week. The strenuous workouts help to relieve tension and keep me in good shape. It's a wonderful outlet for me." Of course, exercising regularly means taking a break from your other responsibilities. Therefore, you may need to ask others to attend to the person with AD in your absence.

To keep a balanced perspective, it is also important for you to engage in recreational or social activities. Whether you do this with or without the person with the disease is a judgment call. Although spending quality time together benefits your relationship, some time away from the person with AD now and then is beneficial for both parties. Attending a sporting event, a play, a movie, a concert, or a party can recharge your batteries. These activities also serve to remind you that providing care for someone is not the only focus of your life and that you deserve to enjoy yourself. And, as stated above, doing something for yourself will also have direct benefits for the person with AD.

It is also important to maintain proper sleeping habits. Although the amount of sleep needed varies from person to person, try to establish a routine that is restful for you. Problems with falling asleep or staying asleep are fairly common and may have many causes such as anxiety, depression, and intake of alcohol and caffeine. Sleep deprivation can have consequences beyond feeling tired and irritable, such as triggering illnesses. It is a good idea to seek professional help if you cannot find a simple solution to a sleep problem. Physicians and others who are sleep specialists can assess and treat the problem.

In spite of your good habits, you may find yourself feeling depressed, angry, or anxious. These feelings may actually get in the way of your eating, exercising, and sleeping properly. Temporarily feeling blue is one matter, but chronically feeling tired, worried, or sad may be a sign of major depression. If you think this may be the case, you should seek professional help, beginning with your physician. Oftentimes the grief associated with caring for a loved one with AD is at the root of depression. Regardless of its underlying causes, depression should be taken seriously and treated promptly. Fortunately, many good treatments for depression are now available, including medications, physical exercise, and talk therapy.

The Importance of Grief

More than forty years ago, Dr. Elisabeth Kübler-Ross described the psychological process of grief experienced by her terminally ill cancer patients in her landmark book, *On Death and Dying.*[2] Her insights led to a better understanding of grief and of the normal stages involved in coming to terms with any type of significant change or loss. You and others caring for someone with AD also face a long series of changes and losses as the disease unfolds. In her memoir, Patti Davis, daughter of President Ronald Reagan, describes her family's experience of caring for him over the course of ten plus years as "the long goodbye."[3] The feelings of grief she describes—helplessness, sadness, disappointment, frustration, despair, and confusion over the losses and changes related to AD—are quite natural. These feelings may be intense from time to time and may threaten to overwhelm you. Ignoring these normal expressions of grief may lead to your becoming stuck in depression, anger, or isolation from others. Physical signs of unresolved grief such as weakness, insomnia, and loss of appetite may also take their toll. This is why reaching out for help is so important. Paying attention to your own grief can help you cope more effectively and adjust to the losses you experience.

According to Dr. Kübler-Ross, grief has certain themes:

Denial. Denial is a natural defense mechanism that helps us to avoid or lessen the impact of a painful event. It is a way of holding onto the past and avoiding current reality. Statements like "I can't believe this is happening" or "This is not such a big deal" or "It can't be Alzheimer's" are all forms of denial. Although denial is a healthy and normal means of coping for a short while, prolonged denial can block the need for action. If the needs of the person with AD are minimized or overlooked, then denial may be harmful. One daughter advises: "The biggest thing is getting over the denial hump. As long as you think that Alzheimer's cannot be identified until autopsy, there is that grain of doubt. You have got to trust the doctor about the diagnosis and then just go ahead and deal with it."

Anger and Depression. Feelings of anger and depression often become noticeable as denial gives way to the reality of loss. Anger may be directed toward God, professionals, family members, or friends. Even worse, anger may be directed to the person with the disease. Anger may also turn inward against yourself, resulting in disturbances of mood or behavior such as social isolation, anxiety, sadness, and depression. Because you are unable to control your circumstances, anger and depression are legitimate responses to your situation. However, there is a danger in allowing these feelings to dominate your thoughts and actions. It is normal to experience these feelings, but they should not linger indefinitely. One husband pointed out: "For me, it was necessary to feel the pain for about three or four months, but after that I had to deal with the fact that I am the main support for this individual. You have to allow yourself to feel the pain at first and then move on to deal with the practical issues of everyday life."

Letting Go. "Moving on" or letting go occurs when anger gives way to more realistic expectations of your situation. You no longer expect the person with the disease to think and act "normally." You begin to adjust your lifestyle to suit the demands of the disease. You realize that the disease is not in your control, and that the future is uncertain. You also no longer insist on imposing your personal wishes on reality and begin to recognize your personal limitations. One wife summed up this view in this way: "Alzheimer's will definitely change your whole life, and your attitude has to change with it. It forces you to consider the other person's needs in front of your own. I can't see it any other way. He doesn't deserve this, and you can't condemn him for it. He can't help what he has, so I have to change my life to support him. It's the agreement we made when we got married."

Acceptance. Acceptance finally occurs when the difficult task of letting go is complete. You no longer wish to return to the past and are able to take each day at a time. Though you may not understand why this disease has come into your life, you accept it as part of your unfolding life story. Acceptance does not mean resignation or defeat, but it means taking life on its own terms. After describing a series of ups and downs in coming to terms with her husband's disease, one woman advised: "Don't be afraid to reach out and get the support you need. Just take each day as it comes and don't try to think too much about the future. If you dwell on how the person may be later on, you won't be able to enjoy their company today."

Bear in mind that you do not pass through these stages of grief all at once. Grief is resolved gradually, sometimes in fits and starts. Some people have described this experience as an "emotional roller coaster." There are too many small, successive changes and losses inherent in AD for you to be able to reach acceptance once and for all. Whenever you attain a measure of acceptance, another incident may occur that may set off another wave of grief. It is important at these trying times not to lose sight of the progress you have already made. Write down any milestones or breakthroughs that you experience so that you can review them when you face a trying time ahead. Having a close relative, friend, counselor, or support group to guide you and remind you of your progress may ease your transition through the normal phases of grief.

Individual and Family Counseling

In the course of caring for a loved one with AD, you may occasionally feel the need for a confidante with whom to share private thoughts and feelings. If the person with AD was your confidante in the past, then someone else must now fill this role, perhaps a close friend or relative. Sometimes a formal relationship with a nonjudgmental and objective outsider, such as a counseling professional, may be preferable.

Counseling is a valuable but often misunderstood resource. One obstacle to counseling is the stigma attached to seeking professional help for personal difficulties. Unfortunately, some people cling to the notion that they must "go it alone" and "be strong" in spite of overwhelming circumstances. Self-sufficiency and privacy are highly regarded values in our culture and can sometimes get in the way of reaching out for help. Yet knowing your limits and recognizing your need for help may actually be a positive step forward in accepting the disease. Potential benefits of engaging in a one-on-one counseling relationship include the following:

- developing better means of handling crisis situations
- addressing your grief reactions
- learning to balance your needs with the needs of the person with AD
- improving your communication with other relatives and friends
- discovering your inner resources for coping in healthy ways
- exploring the use of community resources

Families may also benefit from counseling. Within families caring for a loved one with AD, division of responsibility is rarely fair or equal. Each family member copes in his or her unique way and chooses a measure of responsibility. One person typically assumes the primary role of leader on behalf of the person with AD. Others may help out in a secondary or supportive role. Still others may rarely or never get involved. Differences of opinion about decisions affecting the person with AD are bound to arise. The situation inherently has much potential for conflict, especially if the role of the leader has not been fully accepted by others. One son notes, "I think families have to work hard to stay close when dealing with this disease. In our family, everybody has an opinion about what to do and how to do it." A group meeting, facilitated by a counselor and involving all concerned individuals, may help a family achieve a consensus on key issues.

Spouses and adult children may not be the only ones who are emotionally invested in decisions affecting the person with AD—grandchildren, in-laws, nieces, nephews, and close friends may also have a part to play and should be included in important decisions. One daughter-in-law commented: "My husband and I spend most of our free time looking after his father who has Alzheimer's. My husband's three siblings live nearby but cannot seem to accept what's going on with their father and are minimally involved with him. It took me a long time to get over the resentment I felt toward them." A skilled counselor can facilitate discussion among all concerned parties with the goal of building a consensus. It must be kept in mind that each family has its own unique history and style of handling problems. Old conflicts unrelated to the specific issues presented by AD have a way of reemerging in stressful times, and a counselor can help everyone to focus on current issues as much as possible.

Many types of professionals are trained to provide individual and family counseling. Social workers, psychologists, psychiatrists, nurses, and pastoral counselors are employed in a variety of settings from mental health agencies to churches. They may use different approaches and techniques in helping you and others regain a sense of equilibrium in your lives. Some professionals prefer a traditional, long-term therapy approach, while most others use short-term therapy to focus on solutions to specific issues. Time-limited and problem-focused counseling may be all you need for now.

In choosing a qualified counselor, it is advisable to get a recommendation or to check out credentials. Most professionals engaged in counseling are licensed by the state and accredited through professional organizations. Many counseling services are partially covered by health insurance, and most nonprofit agencies offer a sliding scale for fees. Virtually every county or local community provides financial support to a health or social service agency that offers counseling or makes referrals to counselors in private practice.

Exploring Spiritual Resources

Spirituality may be the least talked about but most commonly explored option among those who have primary responsibility of caring for loved ones with AD. It is in difficult times that questions about faith, hope, and God come into sharp focus:

- "Why is this happening?"
- "Why do bad things happen to good people?"
- "How can God allow this to happen to me? To us?"
- "Is there a God after all?"
- "What does my belief system say about this kind of trial?"

Life's difficulties have a way of intensifying a hunger within us for understanding, strength, and answers to such profound questions. Just as it has been said "There are no atheists in foxholes," spiritual issues often come to the fore among those caring for someone with AD. The search for meaning in the midst of personal confusion seems almost inevitable. For example, in *Tears in God's Bottle,* Wayne Ewing writes from a Christian perspective about how his wife's AD afforded him "an education in the wisdom of the soul."[4] Similarly, in *Ten Thousand Joys and Ten Thousand Sorrows,* Olivia Ames Hoblitzelle uses her Buddhist tradition to reflect positively upon her husband's AD in terms of "the grace of diminishment."[5]

Those unaccustomed to spiritual quests may struggle with preconceived notions about God or the tenets of organized religion. And those who are on a spiritual journey may still feel shaken in their beliefs about and relationship with God. Sharon Fish, whose mother had AD, writes in *Alzheimer's: Caring for Your Loved One, Caring for Yourself,* about her spiritual disillusionment until she sorted out her feelings: "I was very angry with God. My primary support system had always been my church. I stopped going. The Bible has always been my point of strength. I stopped reading. Prayer had always been my source of encouragement. I stopped praying." Yet when tough emotions are addressed in healthy ways, those with a spiritual bent often report an inner peace that helps them persevere with adversity. A woman noted that prayer was a big consolation: "At times, prayer is my only resource, and one that I use quite a bit. Without it, I don't know where I would be today."[6]

Group activities may afford some opportunities for spiritual reflection and growth. The most obvious resources are your church, synagogue, or mosque. If organized religion nurtures your spiritual growth, then worship services involving rituals, traditional prayers, hymns, and other forms of music may be helpful. Small groups may meet regularly to share prayers, discuss faith, and build community. Religious leaders such as ministers, priests, or rabbis are accustomed to addressing spiritual matters and should be consulted for their insight and experience.

Organized religion is not the only arena in which you can explore spirituality. If you are not inclined toward formal religious practice, an attractive alternative may be visiting one of the hundreds of retreat centers that have sprung up in recent years that do not have a strictly religious focus. These centers typically sponsor individual and group programs for spiritual direction and offer workshops on important issues about coping with life. They often employ counselors who serve as spiritual guides, either in the short-term or on an ongoing basis.

If getting away to pursue spiritual affairs is not possible, many solitary activities may also be useful. The following spiritual activities can be pursued alone:

- practicing various types of prayer, rituals, meditation, and yoga
- using books of structured prayers and other spiritual readings
- reflecting on religious scriptures and other traditional writings
- keeping a spiritual journal to record your thoughts and intuitions
- listening to inspirational music
- appreciating the mysteries of nature, art, and sacred objects

Spiritual care alone does not guarantee replenishment of personal energy or a renewed outlook on life. Paying attention to all levels— body, mind, and spirit—is essential for maintaining personal health and wholeness. However, nurturing your inner life can make a positive difference in how you perceive your outer life. Spiritual practices may help you come to terms with AD and lead to a sense of mission in your role. One man caring for his wife summarized his new point of view:

> I used to think that if you did right, then happiness would follow. But then Alzheimer's came along and blew that away. I guess God had different plans, so I needed to learn how to make the best of a bad situation. I can't say that I've got this disease down pat, but it's not as hard as I thought it could be. My wife can still do a lot of things for herself, and she doesn't mind my help. So we are just taking one day at a time.

Keeping a Journal

There are now dozens of books based on the diaries of those who have cared for relatives with AD. These husbands, wives, sons, and daughters did not begin writing with the goal of publishing. On the contrary, their daily writings served as outlets for their thoughts and feelings about coping with the disease. The personal practice of "journaling" enabled them to reflect on their experiences and to gain a better perspective on their situation.

AD invariably evokes many strong feelings, and keeping such feelings bottled up inside is unhealthy. You, too, might find it helpful to keep a running account of your personal reactions to the different stages of AD in a diary or private journal. No writing experience is required, since keeping a journal is purely an exercise in becoming more aware of your thoughts and feelings and a way to unclutter your mind. Writing also allows both your dark and light sides to become better known. When you chart your course during a stressful or confusing time, patterns typically emerge that can help lead you to self-discovery and solutions to problems. Your written record of experiences may also serve as reminders of past pitfalls to be avoided and successes to be savored.

Since keeping a journal requires some discipline, here are a few simple guidelines:

- A journal's most valuable quality is its flexibility. It is important to make it your own forum for self-expression. Let your inhibitions down and do not edit yourself. This is your private project and no one else's business. Add doodles, sketches, and art to suit your mood.

- Where and when you write must fit into your lifestyle. If you can write during periods of stress, then do so. If not, wait for when you feel less distracted.

- The tools you use do not matter as long as they are right for you. Use a pen, pencil, spiral notebook, typewriter, or computer—whatever works for you. Keep things simple to make writing as easy and satisfying as possible.

- Beginning the process is probably the biggest step. Keeping a journal may develop into a pleasurable routine after a month or two. Ten minutes a day may be a good place to start.

Maintaining a Sense of Humor

Numerous studies have shown that humor can go a long way toward alleviating stress. Good fun, laughter, and play are effective tools in coping with the pressures of caring for someone with AD. You may think, "What's so funny about Alzheimer's?" and this is a fair question to ask, since, on many levels, it's no laughing matter. But much of the distress associated with a situation is related to how it is perceived. Taking a lighthearted view can alter the meaning of a situation and make all the difference in coping. A woman I know named Juanita Tucker explains her need to see the brighter side in relation to her husband's AD:

> I have gone through days filled with concern and confusion as well as aggravation and anger. But I have learned to be flexible, to sort out what is really important, to keep my sense of humor. For example, one evening I was so insistent that Allan put on his

pajamas at bedtime. "One doesn't sleep in shorts and a T-shirt!" I said. With a look of resignation, he finally put on his pajamas. He then looked at me with a puzzled expression and asked, in all seriousness, "Is this written down somewhere?" One's priorities do have a way of changing after these funny encounters.[7]

A man I know, whose wife has AD, constantly tells jokes as a way of easing tension. He once remarked, "My wife has gotten preoccupied with the hereafter since she developed this disease."

"How so?" I asked.

"Well," he said, "whenever she walks into a room, she'll stand there a minute, then say 'What am I here after?'"

Such humor may not appeal to everyone, but it seems to work well for him.

It is also important to spend time with friends who remind you not to get completely caught up in your troubles and to laugh now and then. One woman notes, "I have a group of lady friends that has socialized together for more than thirty years. Those women remind me how to laugh, even when I'm feeling down about my husband having Alzheimer's." In support groups for the relatives and friends of people with AD, a topic discussed in the next chapter, humor is a staple of virtually every meeting.

. . . .

There is a child within each of us who can remember how to enjoy life under any circumstances. It takes a conscious choice to seek this perspective. When Gail Sheehy was doing background work for her best-selling book, *Pathfinders,* she discovered that the ability to see humor in difficult situations was a primary way for people to cope with change and uncertainty. She referred to those who could successfully deal with life's crises as "pathfinders." In a real sense, family members and friends who learn to navigate the challenges of AD are pathfinders, too. While it is important to cut your own path, do yourself the favor of calling upon others to help you manage your self-care.

As the disease progresses, increasing amounts of time and energy will be required of you and others in caring for the person with AD. As the leading care partner, you may be especially vulnerable to the worry that comes with this major responsibility. You must take steps to care for yourself to remain physically, mentally, and spiritually strong over the long haul. It will sometimes be necessary to call on outside sources for help so that you can nurture yourself regularly. In the next chapter I will address some forms of help that you may need in the future, as the disease progresses.

12 Obtaining the Help You May Need

*We have prepared for the worst, and now
we are planning to live expecting the best.
If the worst comes, we are ready for it. If it doesn't,
we will have not wasted today worrying about it.*

Betty Davis, noted in her husband's memoir,
My Journey into Alzheimer's Disease

It is possible that the early stages of AD may last for many years—or the disease may progress more quickly. You cannot be sure what the future holds, and preparing for every contingency is both practically unrealistic and emotionally draining. It is helpful to an extent to learn what might happen over the next three to five years. At the same time, you cannot allow yourself to feel overwhelmed by potential care issues in the future. It is impossible for you to imagine how you might feel and think then. This chapter focuses first on services you might need in the near term and then addresses the usual progression of AD. This book does not address issues related to the later stages of the disease. Numerous other books, pamphlets, websites, and videos cover more-advanced care issues.

Enlisting Help

Nearly everyone involved in directly caring for someone with AD feels the need for help at one point or another. You should not aim to be an exception—no medals are awarded to those who struggle alone. It is not a sign of failure or inadequacy for you to seek outside help. On the contrary, it may be a sign of personal strength to recognize your limits and get the help you need and deserve. Caring for someone does not automatically mean that you alone will directly provide care at all times. That solo approach had been tried and failed by countless others in a similar situation. Your commitment to someone with AD entails ensuring a good quality of life by all available means, regardless of who is actually providing the care. Therefore, you should always feel free to call upon other people and services for assistance, as long as you retain overall responsibility or share it with others.

In this sense, it may be useful to consider yourself as a care manager, instead of a care provider. A simple definition of management is "getting things done through other people." It is important to enlist the help of others and delegate responsibilities whenever possible. This typically means calling upon relatives, friends, and neighbors for help. If those informal resources are unavailable or prove insufficient, you need to consider other forms of help. Such resources worth considering are support groups, in-home care, and adult day services.

Participating in a Support Group

Chapter 10 discussed the potential benefits of support groups for people in the early stage of AD. Support groups for relatives and friends can also be helpful but most groups are not limited to early stages issues. For the most part these groups attract people dealing with the middle and late stages of AD. For this reason, participating in a support group may have limited value for you unless the group's leader makes an effort to balance the needs of all members. If at all possible, join a group specifically for people dealing with the early stages or encourage a local organization to form one.

Support groups serve two basic purposes. First, they aim to educate families and friends about the many aspects of AD. Second, they enable members to offer emotional support to one another. Most support groups consist of between eight and twenty people and are led by a health-care professional or an experienced family member. The group leader is responsible for facilitating, keeping order, and focusing on the needs for education and emotional support. Meetings ordinarily last about one and one-half hours and are held monthly. Membership is usually free, and members can drop in and out at will. Some groups are structured with specific goals and agendas in mind, but most groups are conducted in an informal, conversational style.

A self-help philosophy is central to most support groups. Members have a chance to share their collective wisdom by exchanging stories about caring for someone with AD. The operating principle is that one single perspective on the disease is less helpful than having the different perspectives of many experienced people. Members also share information about the symptoms of AD, how to handle communication difficulties, and how to find appropriate forms of help such as paid companions, adult day centers, or residential care. Outside speakers are occasionally invited to address specific topics of interest such as legal and financial planning or issues related to intimacy and sexuality.

Some topics discussed in support groups may be premature for newcomers to the disease. Stories about potential symptoms and experiences may be distressing to those caring for someone in the early stages of AD. Nevertheless, an effective group leader protects newcomers against undue worry about the future. The knowledge, experience, and skill of leaders can vary from group to group. If you do not receive the help you need after a meeting or two, consider joining another group or returning to the group later.

Learning about the disease in a support group does not take place only on an intellectual level. Rather, sharing feelings in a safe and confidential atmosphere enables members to realize that they are not alone. All thoughts and feelings are fair game for discussion in a group, which can be a liberating experience for those who feel lost and alone. You can freely discuss the dilemma of caring for someone with AD while caring for yourself without guilt, embarrassment, or criticism. You may get a great deal of comfort and hope from meeting others who are coping well under similar circumstances. One daughter observed: "It's important to find other people to talk to about the various problems of the disease. It's also good to get help in learning how to be more patient and understanding with the person who has the Alzheimer's."

Because of the range of different needs and circumstances of those who care for people with AD, many specialized support groups have sprung up. For example, some groups are geared exclusively to spouses, and other groups are just for adult children. As noted, groups devoted specifically to the early stages of the disease may also be available. These specialized groups enable participants to establish rapport quickly by virtue of their similar concerns.

Although support groups alone cannot give you all the education and emotional support needed to deal with AD, they can be a valuable source of help. Indeed, support groups have proven to be a real lifeline for some individuals and families. Those who lack a solid network of relatives and friends may find a compassionate circle of people "in the same boat." To find out about support groups in your area, contact the local chapter of the Alzheimer's Association (www.alz.org or 800-272-3900) or the Alzheimer Society of Canada (www.alzheimer.ca or 416-488-8772). Many hospitals, adult day centers, and social-service agencies also sponsor support groups.

For those who cannot or do not wish to venture into traditional support groups, technology now affords a way to be in contact with others without leaving your home. Many nonprofit organizations and commercial enterprises have formed online groups and message boards to help people with common interests to communicate easily with one another. The above organizations, the Alzheimer's Foundation of America (www.alzfdn.org or 866-232-8484), and other organizations focused on related brain diseases sponsor online groups and message boards (see Additional Resources at the end of this book).

Using Help at Home

At first, most people in the early stages of the disease can be left home alone without much worry about their well-being and safety. However, you or your loved one with AD will gradually begin to wonder if being alone is a good idea. There may be growing limits to his or her ability to be self-directed and feel comfortable at home alone. You will eventually realize that supervision is needed some of the time, and then ultimately at all times, in order to reduce worry—yours and your loved one's. Whether such help is needed on a part-time, full-time, or live-in basis is primarily your decision and will depend on many factors, including affordability. It is not realistic for you to be available on a continuous basis, twenty-four hours a day, seven days a week. Nobody can handle all the responsibilities involved in caring for someone with AD alone, nor should such heroics be attempted. If care is to continue indefinitely at home, it will be necessary for you to get regular breaks.

It takes courage to reach out, but you and your loved one with AD stand to benefit from the help of other people. You may initially prefer to call upon your relatives, neighbors, and friends. They may fill in gaps or be available on a regular basis, but you must overcome a natural tendency to believe that they will somehow just understand what is needed and when it is needed. You may need to assert yourself and ask for specific types of assistance at specific times. Even with the help of one or more supportive persons, you may need to consider hiring additional help. You may be able to work out a paid arrangement with someone you know so that the helper's personal commitment is bolstered by a financial incentive. Do not hesitate to consider such a business proposition with someone you know, since the alternative of hiring someone through an agency can be risky. Volunteer services may also be available in some areas, so this avenue should be explored. Many religious congregations have formed groups of volunteer or "ministers of care" to assist individuals and families.

Bringing a stranger into the home to care for the person with AD can be a big gamble, so this option is usually not considered until it becomes essential. Worries about having an outsider in the home cannot be easily dismissed. When you are the chief provider of care, you can count on your own reliability, sensitivity, and honesty. As soon as you share responsibility with others, especially a paid helper, these concerns can no longer be guaranteed. Myriad troubling questions arise. Will the helper show up on time? Will he or she be patient and kind? Might she or he be trustworthy, patronizing, or worse, a thief? Yet although there are risks involved in bringing a paid helper into the home, the risks of not getting help may be even bigger. And there may be unexpected benefits if you hire someone who meets or exceeds your expectations. This kind of arrangement can prove successful for everyone if the right person is found for the job.

You can hire someone either privately or through a home-care agency, and either approach has advantages and disadvantages. On the one hand, you benefit by having a direct choice instead of settling for whoever is sent by an agency. You can be selective and set your own standards. The expense of a private arrangement is also far less than using an agency. You can negotiate an hourly, daily, or weekly rate rather than paying a higher rate set by an agency. On the other hand, there are also several drawbacks to a private arrangement. Unemployment, Social Security, and Medicare taxes are supposed to be paid on behalf of your employee if payments exceed one thousand dollars a year. If a paid helper gets sick or quits, you are not guaranteed an instant replacement.

Home-care agencies provide an array of services on a fee-for-service basis and offer several levels of staff. A "companion," homemaker, or nursing assistant, may be well-suited to providing most services you need. Turnover tends to be a big problem at home-care agencies as well as in private arrangements. However, an agency can usually provide a substitute or replacement within a short time. The challenges of screening, interviewing, and hiring the right person may outweigh the financial benefits. Yet there is no guarantee that someone hired through an agency will be any better qualified than someone you hire privately.

The cost of home care is not paid by Medicare or other forms of insurance. The exception is long-term care insurance, and a claim must be filed and approved by the insurance company. As a result, out-of-pocket expenses can be quite high. Rates range from $15 to $25 an hour up to $250 for one entire day. As noted in Chapter 9, the cost of hiring someone to perform medical, maintenance, and personal-care services should qualify as an itemized tax deduction under federal law, provided that all medical expenses exceed 7.5 percent of adjusted gross income in a given year. Whether the services are considered "medical" depends on the nature of the services performed and not on the qualifications of the person performing them. If a paid helper performs both medical and housekeeping services such as dressing, grooming, and bathing, only the medical portion is considered tax deductible. If the expense of hiring someone does not qualify as medical care as defined by the Internal Revenue Service, it may still qualify for the Household and Dependent Care Credit if the person with AD resides with you.

Government subsidies for services provided by home-care agencies under contract with state-funded programs might be available to people with low incomes and assets. Contact the Eldercare Locator at www.eldercare.gov or (800) 677-1116 for further information about programs and eligibility requirements in your area.

Although cost is an important consideration, distrust of strangers and concern about the quality of care are the most common barriers to using in-home services. You can take several steps to ensure that risks are kept to a minimum when working with an agency:

Identify needs. What types of services are needed—companionship, meal preparation, dressing, bathing? A job description that fits the particular needs of the person with AD should be written down and discussed with a prospective agency or employee. If you want your loved one to be an active participant in activities with a paid helper or a passive recipient of services, then the nature of the job should be clarified. Also, a schedule showing the days and hours that you need covered in a given week should be organized. Home-care agencies usually require that you hire a helper for a minimum of four hours a day. If you are uncertain about how often to have your helper come, at least twice a week is a good start.

Make your own selection of an agency and helper. Obtain a list of agencies that are known to specialize in caring for people with AD. Ask for referrals from the local chapter of the Alzheimer's Association, the state agency on aging, or discharge planners at nearby hospitals. A good agency promptly returns calls, carefully listens to requests, and provides written details about services and costs. You should discuss your specific needs and expectations with the agency and the paid helper since it cannot be assumed that the agency has communicated details to the helper. If possible, conduct an interview with the prospective helper to inquire about his or her training, experience, and references. A background check of past criminal history should also be done by the agency. Above all, look for personal qualities such as patience, understanding, a sense of humor, and good personal chemistry with your loved one with AD.

Develop a working relationship with the helper. A paid helper deserves to be given clear instructions and immediate feedback, both positive and negative. Pass along the benefits of your experience by teaching the helper what works and what doesn't work in relation to your loved one with AD. Make concrete suggestions, provide encouragement, and ask clarifying questions. Consider sharing educational resources with your helper to increase his or her knowledge about the disease. It may take several visits by the helper before everyone involved settles into a routine.

Evaluate progress. Evaluation should be an ongoing process, but regular times need to be set aside for discussing your concerns. Reward good work and address any problems in a straightforward manner. Difficulties are inevitable, but good communication can minimize them and yield quick solutions. Flagrant mistakes and repeated misunderstandings call for intervention by the paid helper's supervisor.

Choosing an Adult Day Center

Another option to consider is an adult day center, a community-based program offering therapeutic activities and individualized services in a group setting for older adults with a variety of disabilities. Most people who attend adult day centers have AD, typically in the middle and late stages, and other people may have other medical conditions such as Parkinson's disease or are stroke affected. As noted earlier in Chapter 8, a growing number of adult day centers have specialized programs for people in the early stages of AD or mild cognitive impairment (MCI). Sometimes these places are referred to as *adult day-care centers,* a term that can be offensive to someone with AD because of its association with young children. Using terms such as *day center* or *club* may be more appealing to someone who rightfully does not wish to be treated like a child.

Those attending adult day centers participate in structured activities under the direction of a professional team. These activities may be physical, recreational, and intellectual in nature and often involve the creative arts such as music and art. The daily schedule of activities includes nutritious meals and snacks. At some places, participants prepare these foods as part of the activities program. Some centers also provide transportation, dispense medications, and assist with personal tasks such as bathing. People with AD typically enjoy the opportunity to be with other people in a place where their needs and abilities are understood.

Adult day centers may be a good option to consider when one or more of the conditions listed below are present. The person with AD:

- appears unable to provide him- or herself with any structure for daily activities
- is isolated from others for more than a few hours a day and misses companionship
- cannot be safely left alone at home
- lives with someone who works outside the home or needs regular time away from home for other reasons

The decision to involve someone with AD in an adult day center includes several considerations. First and foremost, you must be comfortable with the idea. You may imagine that the person with AD would probably not like it, but you need to keep an open mind. Staff members at these centers usually welcome exploratory visits, and you may be pleasantly surprised at their friendliness and expertise. Two daughters reluctantly brought their mother to a center one day, convinced that she would reject the idea of participation upon an introductory visit. They claimed that she had never been a "joiner" and was too proud to be around others with memory problems. While the daughters met with one staff member, other staff invited their mother into a group activity. When they reunited an hour later, the daughters were surprised by their mother's reaction: "I like this place. The people here are forgetful like me, and yet nobody is expected to remember. They have nice people here who help keep you on track."

When discussing this option with the person with AD, it is best to use a positive, calm, and reassuring manner. Simple and brief explanations, such as, "It's a place where you can meet some friendly people" or "The doctor thinks you should try this out, so I think it's worth checking out, too" are most effective. Most people with AD will follow this type of suggestion if you set the right tone from the beginning. Some people with AD, like the mother mentioned above, react well to their first visit to an adult day center; others are put off by the unfamiliar situation. Staff members at these centers have a lot of experience with this and know how to ease the adjustment. Some places have a staff member conduct home visits to get to know prospective participants. It is customary to try out the adult day center two or three times a week at first and then to increase the frequency of visits as the person's comfort level grows. Although the person with AD may express some resistance initially, allow the trial to continue for a few weeks. The payoff comes when he or she begins to enjoy the company of other participants and staff.

Most centers are open five days a week, and some are open on Saturdays as well. The cost is roughly $70 a day. In the United States, Medicare does not cover the cost, so most people have to pay out of their own pocket. However, the cost should qualify as an itemized tax deduction for medical expenses under federal law, provided that all medical expenses exceed 7.5 percent of adjusted gross income in a given year. Again, if the expense does not qualify for this type of tax deduction, it may still qualify for the Household and Dependent Care Credit if the person with AD resides with you. Financial assistance for those with low incomes and assets may be available through public sources such as the state Department on Aging or the U.S. Department of Veterans Affairs. A sliding-fee scale may also be available at some centers for those people ineligible for subsidies. Discounts are usually allowed for people who attend daily.

Information about local adult day centers can be obtained through a hospital, clinic, home-care agency, social-service agency, senior center, or a professional geriatric-care manager. Again, a list of centers is available through the National Adult Day Services Association (www.nadsa.org or 877-745-1440) and the Eldercare Locator (www.eldercare.gov or 800-677-1116).

The National Family Caregiver Support Program

The U.S. government funds the National Family Caregiver Support Program to assist families who care for older disabled adults, including those with AD. Whether or not you consider yourself to be a caregiver, this program may benefit you now or in the future. The national program is administered locally by private, nonprofit organizations or government entities known as area agencies on aging (AAAs), which contract with community-service providers to offer the following five basic services:

1. information about available services

2. assistance in gaining access to supportive services

3. individual counseling, organization of support groups, and training to assist caregivers in making decisions and solving problems

4. respite care to enable caregivers to be temporarily relieved from caregiving responsibilities

5. supplemental services to complement the care provided by caregivers

The local AAA should be among the first resources that you contact for information about these and other useful services. Priority consideration is given to persons in the greatest social and economic need, but the program has no income or asset limits for eligibility. You can also find out about services in your local area by contacting the Eldercare Locator.

Learning More About AD

The challenges of the disease right now may be more than enough for you to handle without worrying about the future, yet you may be curious about what may lie ahead. If current challenges are handled well, your self-confidence will certainly grow as you face the future. Exercise caution in anticipating these changes, though, since planning for every contingency is not possible. Nevertheless, you and others involved in day-to-day responsibilities should have some idea of the changes that accompany AD, so that you can prepare accordingly.

Now is the time, in the early stages, for you and others involved in the care of someone with AD to learn how to pace yourselves and to prepare for the long haul. Caring for someone with AD is analogous to running a marathon. Sprinting from the start will ruin your chances of completing the long race, and so pacing yourself is necessary. For example, some family members and friends panic upon hearing the diagnosis of AD, project their worst fears, and imagine a dire future. Such emotions are understandable but are not helpful and may cause you to become unduly worried or sad. Other people may eagerly absorb whatever information they can read about the disease. Although gaining knowledge is important, drowning yourself in information can be counterproductive.

Table 12.1 on the next page gives an overview of typical symptoms at the early, middle, and late stages of AD. Note that these three stages are not clear-cut, and symptoms frequently overlap. The continuum from complete independence to total dependence may take anywhere from three to ten or more years. Most people can be cared for at home for the major part of the disease, and relocating them to a residential care facility is not inevitable. Many people with AD live at home with lots of support until the end of life. Furthermore, many people with AD never reach the late stages of the disease but die from other illnesses before reaching a point of total dependence. As symptoms worsen, the amount of help needed by the person with the disease will increase accordingly.

Generally speaking, the more troubling symptoms that sometimes occur in the later stages of AD are the ones that receive the most attention in popular descriptions of the disease. The media tend to focus on worst-case scenarios. However, problems such as aggressive behavior, wandering, hallucinations, insomnia, and incontinence do not occur in all cases. The disease does not include an "angry stage," as has been stereotyped to be part of the process. If and when such problems occur, they may be triggered by many causes, such as a drug reaction, a pain-related condition, or an acute illness such as a urinary tract infection. Unpleasant behaviors are often responses to disturbing acts and words of insensitive or distressed care providers. These behaviors seriously affect the quality of life for everyone directly involved and deserve careful assessment and creative responses. Do not hesitate to call upon professionals for help if these problems arise.

Table 12.1. The Symptoms and Stages of Alzheimer's Disease

Brain Function	Early Stage	Middle Stage	Late Stage
Memory	Shows loss of recent memory much of the time; repeats oneself	Shows more-consistent loss of recent memory and some long-term memories	Mixes up the past and the present; may "time travel" to an earlier period of life
Language	Has trouble finding words and keeping track of conversations	Has more trouble completing sentences and understanding others	Shows severe difficulty expressing and understanding words
Orientation	May get lost in unfamiliar places and loses track of time, dates	May get lost in familiar places and may not know the season, day, or year	Has trouble identifying familiar people and places
Coordination skills	Has trouble writing and using familiar objects	Has difficulty coordinating hands and legs	May have trouble walking and can be at risk for falls
Mood or behavior	May appear withdrawn, apathetic, depressed, or irritable	May appear more withdrawn, depressed, irritable, or agitated	May experience agitation, hallucinations, or delusions
Daily tasks	Needs reminders with household tasks	Cannot do most household tasks and needs reminders and help with personal care tasks	Needs help with nearly all tasks

Note: Symptoms vary from person to person, and symptoms may overlap between stages.

Most people with AD will die from other medical causes such as heart disease, cancer, or a stroke before they reach the late stages of the disease. It can be said that these people die *with* AD, not because of it. However, if someone survives to the late stages, the possibility exists that he or she may die *because* of AD. In the final stage of the disease, people often lose the ability to walk and talk, and they develop problems with chewing and swallowing. At this point, pneumonia usually occurs and triggers death. For anyone facing the final weeks and months of life, regardless of diagnosis, hospice is a service aimed at providing care and comfort to both terminally ill individuals and their families.

Hospice involves a team of health-care professionals and trained volunteers who deliver care wherever people live—home, assisted-living facility, or nursing home. Some hospice organizations also offer special homes or facilities where people can rest comfortably in their final days or weeks. Hospice services and necessary medical equipment are paid for by all health-insurance companies, mainly because of the ability of hospices to avoid costly and unnecessary hospitalizations. Keep hospice in mind if at some point you believe that someone is facing the end of life, whether due to AD or another condition. A physician or another health-care provider can offer guidance, and you may also contact a hospice directly to discuss a referral. To learn more about end-of-life care and to locate a hospice in your area, contact Caring Connections (www.caringinfo.org or 800-658-8898).

Over the past decade, both professionals and family members of people with AD have produced a virtual flood of information about AD. Some of the more helpful resources are listed at the end of this book. Books, pamphlets, websites, and videos abound, but the quality of information varies widely. The tone in some materials is rather negative and frightening in that these materials have a tendency to dwell on the growing inability of the person with AD and the burden on families. Grim images of individuals and families struggling to survive the "funeral that never ends" can be misleading and depressing. It takes a discerning mind to hear and read about the gamut of possibilities and not feel overwhelmed. Seek reliable and balanced information. Certainly many pessimistic stories are out there, but you can also find many positive stories, too, about hope, love, and meaning associated with caring for someone with AD. Stay informed but do not give up on the goal of achieving a good quality of life for everyone involved.

Another disadvantage of the plethora of information on topics such as diagnosis, genetics, treatments, alternative medicine, and coping strategies for AD is that you may become overwhelmed. The bottom line message here is to become informed as needed instead of trying to learn everything at once. One woman shared wisdom based on experience: "At first I tried to get my hands on everything about this disease, but I ended up getting more confused and upset. Now I advise others to stop reading about Alzheimer's and start coping day-by-day. I know this approach has worked for me."

. . . .

Your own expectations for finding enjoyment in life, now and in the future, will naturally be tempered by your loved one's disease, but keep in mind that personal fulfillment and meaning are still possible. A positive outlook is possible. It is a choice. Valuing each day and living in the moment may become part of a "new normal." Making life as enjoyable as possible may take on new meaning when you consider that time is running out for the person with the disease to enjoy activities in customary ways. Take opportunities to enjoy your time together now, since the disease gradually changes those who are affected. Everett Jordan reflected on this sense of "borrowed time" with his wife with AD in an educational video: "I know this time together with Betty is not going to last. So I want to make the most of our remaining time together. Whether we have just one tomorrow, a hundred tomorrows, or a thousand tomorrows, I want to make each day as meaningful as possible for her."[1]

Changing your attitude and behavior to accommodate the presence of AD in your life doesn't happen overnight. Nothing less than major lifestyle changes are called for, a process that takes time. Along the way, your adjustment process may feel painstakingly slow. Mistakes are inevitable in the course of learning how to cope effectively with your changing roles and responsibilities. Do not be discouraged by setbacks. Such disappointments are also opportunities to learn new skills and redefine what constitutes a good life.

A wise woman whose husband had AD once told me, "The human spirit is like a tea bag: You don't know your own strength until you've been in hot water." AD will certainly test you in all kinds of ways. Although the disease cannot be stopped or reversed, you will always have the freedom to choose how you cope with its challenges. May you discover surprising strength within your own spirit.

13 Voices of Experience

As we cultivate peace and happiness in ourselves,
we also nourish peace and happiness in those we love.
Thich Nhat Hanh

It has been said that experience is the mother of wisdom. It is true that many important life lessons can be learned from experience, but there is no guarantee. Likewise, much knowledge and wisdom can come from people who have already completed the journey of AD, and relatives and friends of people with the disease have written dozens of books. Every story is unique and reflects the personality and perception of each author. Many of these books depict the experience of caring for someone with AD in bleak terms, whereas others offer good guidance and a positive tone. The same can be said of websites. Be careful about which materials you read or recommend to others. Some of the better ones have been listed in the Notes and Resources sections at the back of this book.

This chapter highlights the experience of family members and friends of people with AD who completed a survey that I developed specifically for this chapter. I wanted to hear directly from those who have cared for loved ones with AD so you could learn from them. The survey was sent to them with the cooperation of my professional colleagues working at AD research centers and other AD service programs throughout the United States and Canada. Within a month, I received nearly two hundred replies from husbands, wives, sons, daughters, daughters-in-law, sons-in-laws, siblings, and close friends of people who have had AD. Their combined experience caring for someone with AD totals over 1,400 years, which is an average of seven years per person since the diagnosis. Virtually all of these care partners had loved ones who had already advanced into the later stages of the disease. I did not inquire about their racial, ethnic, and cultural backgrounds, so they are not necessarily a representative group. Your experience may or may not be represented by them, although some of their thoughts and feelings may parallel your own. I think they have much wisdom to share.

While some individuals offered short, simple responses to a series of open-ended questions, others wrote lengthy explanations and anecdotes. Some people wrote in straightforward, factual terms, but most told of an emotion-filled experience, often referred to as a "journey." Most were either older individuals themselves or were middle-aged people caring for older people. In a few cases, the individuals with AD were middle-aged, and their spouses were respondents. Most people are still caring for someone at home, some care for others who now live in residential care facilities, and a few had experienced the death of a loved one with AD within the past year. Whereas some clearly appear angry and depressed, most have reached a measure of hard-fought acceptance. Their similarities and differences will be illustrated through a question-and-answer format.

Questions and Answers

Q: *When you first heard the diagnosis of Alzheimer's disease, what was your initial reaction? How did your thoughts and feelings about the disease change over time?*

About half of the people report that the diagnosis was a total shock. Feelings of denial, disbelief, anger, fear, and sadness were common at first. The notion of AD as "the worst possible disease" was a typical reaction to the news. One woman writes, "Upon hearing the diagnosis, I thought my whole world would fall apart. It felt as if my husband had been handed a death sentence."

A few people say they ignored the diagnosis, not talking about it or doing anything in response for weeks or months afterward. A wife writes, "After a few weeks, I collected my senses and began to rearrange our future plans." Getting the proper information and support generally enabled them to cope with difficult feelings and develop positive coping strategies. A husband notes, "At first I was devastated. For about six months, we did nothing in response. After a respectful period of pondering, we got involved in research projects, support groups, and many other activities related to Alzheimer's." Getting a realistic understanding about the nature of AD was essential for coping with the shock experienced at the beginning. A son writes, "Since I have a close friend whose mother is in the late stages of Alzheimer's, I was horrified contemplating Mom's future. But then I began to realize that it can be a lengthy process and people can function pretty well for a long time. I switched my attitude and found ways to help her."

For the other half of people who had expected to hear the diagnosis was AD, an evaluation confirmed what they already had suspected for months or years beforehand. For many of these individuals, the label "Alzheimer's disease" offered insight into the symptoms and provided a framework for better understanding. A wife writes, "At least I finally knew what was causing his unusual behavior and could learn how to make adjustments." The diagnosis also enabled them to talk openly about the disease and to be proactive about decisions that needed to be made. A daughter writes, "It was sad to know that my mother had struggled with this alone prior to being diagnosed. We knew something was wrong but pretended it would go away. The diagnosis gave us a way to bring it out into the open."

Although some people report being intellectually prepared to hear the diagnosis, it nevertheless evoked grief as feelings turned to loss and worry about a loved one's decline. Again, the implications of the diagnosis were generally unknown, and most respondents could imagine only a dreadful future. A daughter writes, "Over time, we've come to understand the implications and impact of the disease on both our family and my mother." A wife notes, "It was helpful to know that it is a disease which, though predictable in many ways, is very individual in the way it alters the person's thinking and behavior. I learned to be observant as to how it affected [my husband] specifically, and that helped me determine how to help him."

Q: *At the time of diagnosis, did the doctor or another professional say or do anything particularly helpful or unhelpful?*

Several people report that obtaining a proper evaluation and diagnosis from a physician was in itself a major struggle. Their complaints about a loved one's poor memory were often unheeded or attributed simply to "old age." A couple of people recall being dismissed by physicians who coldly remarked that nothing could be done about memory loss. A woman reflects back on that time: "I am still angry about the doctor's pessimism. I have since learned that there is so much you can do, and little of it has to do with medicine." Other people report getting only a vague diagnosis at first and their lingering uncertainty about the condition proved frustrating. On the other hand, many people tell of getting proper yet incomplete attention from physicians. Seldom were they encouraged to obtain a second opinion or seek out a professional well versed in caring for someone with AD. If dissatisfied with a primary-care physician, specialists were typically sought out and found to be good sources of help.

Physicians were generally knowledgeable about medications for AD. A prescription was usually written for one of the AD drugs, and potential benefits and side effects were briefly discussed. Medical issues were addressed, but the myriad social and emotional aspects of the disease were ignored for the most part. One woman complained that although the doctor called her adult son to discuss the diagnosis, her key role as a spouse of someone with AD was overlooked. In most cases, the impact of the disease on relatives and friends was not foremost in physicians' minds.

Apart from those physicians at memory disorder clinics or AD research centers, very few physicians offered to convene a meeting of concerned relatives and friends. In those special cases, physicians answered questions, shared printed materials, and made referrals to community resources. Family members share universal appreciation for straight facts, realistic advice, and warm concern. A daughter-in-law reflects, "The doctor made a point of saying that there was life after a diagnosis. That positive message has stayed with our family and has challenged us to make the most of the situation."

Q: *As you look back at the time of the diagnosis, what would have been more helpful?*

Some people report satisfaction with physicians, but most expressed concern that physicians did not adequately prepare them for either the short-term or long-term consequences of AD. A wife notes, "I would have benefited from more aggressive follow-up. I got the impression that a one-shot consultation was the doctor's modus operandi." Family members did not expect physicians to address all of their issues and were relatively forgiving because of the physician's busy schedule. At the same time, they clearly needed ongoing support, education, and services and were generally not directed to resources. One husband observes, "Physicians know little about the day-to-day care of people with this disease. I had to make do on my own until I got connected to the right people." To help him cope with his wife's condition, he found a social worker, a financial advisor, an attorney, and a support group. A wife says simply, "Above all, I needed reassurance that all was not lost."

A daughter-in-law writes, "What our family needed was a learning environment. A multidisciplinary team would have been most helpful, but I would have settled for just one mentor. It's tough to learn things on your own when you don't even know the right questions to ask." Lack of information appears to compound feelings of loneliness and desperation. A husband notes, "Having come through this initial period, I believe there is a big need to acknowledge the emotional trauma and get guidance in taking on a new role."

In light of many disappointing remarks about physicians, it is interesting to note that several research studies that have explored physician and family interactions have yielded similar findings. Families facing the diagnosis of AD generally consider care by physicians to be less than ideal. Families consistently complain that physicians give little attention to their need for information and referral and seldom address emotional distress. Unfortunately, both family members and diagnosed individuals express widespread dissatisfaction about interactions with health-care professionals. In response, a group of people in the early stages of AD met under the auspices of the Alzheimer's

Association and in 2009 published eleven "Principles for a Dignified Diagnosis" that begins with a simple one: "Talk to me, the person with dementia."[1]

Ongoing support, education, and services are needed throughout the course of the disease. Setting the right tone for the future may be the best form of help provided by physicians or other health professionals at the outset. At the same time, families must seek out additional forms of help instead of relying solely upon a single health-care professional to address their needs.

Q: *How have relatives, friends, neighbors, and others reacted to the news that someone they know has been diagnosed with Alzheimer's disease?*

Nearly all of the family members report a mixed bag—favorable reactions by some people and unfavorable reactions by others. They tell of varied reactions of acceptance and denial among relatives and friends. Some people were already aware that something was amiss, many months or, in some cases, years before the actual diagnosis. Others were completely surprised and required more time to come to terms, especially if they were not close to the situation. A spouse recalls, "At first, most friends were uncomfortable with the changes in him, and I found myself in the middle as an 'interpreter.' A few chose not to see him as he had become, preferring instead to remember him the way he was." Many people agree that other relatives and friends tend to withdraw. Several individuals agree that, "You find out who your friends are." Older spouses, in particular, report feeling sadness in seeing friends drift away in these trying times.

Despite such disappointments, many other individuals report that some relatives and friends manage to rise to the occasion and help out in significant ways. A woman says, "It has been gratifying to see how many people really care about us. I don't know what I would do without such a strong network of supporters." One man says he is grateful that he and his wife with AD are still treated as a couple by their friends. He notes, "They have adapted to the changes better than I had anticipated."

Q: *If experienced, what is your opinion of current medications used in treating the disease?*

The majority of respondents report experience in having loved ones use one or more of AD drugs. Although some indicate that side effects were intolerable, most comment favorably. At the same time, they are quick to point out that miracles are not to be expected. They caution that there is no way of really knowing if a drug is working or if the person would be the same without taking it. Most had observed an initial improvement in "alertness" or "initiative," but such benefits tapered off. If one particular drug did not seem effective or caused adverse effects, another drug was usually tried. Drugs seem to offer hope that something is being done to improve symptoms or slow the progression of AD. Several people note their concern that if an AD drug was discontinued, decline might result that might not have otherwise occurred.

Whether or not a medication was effective, most people believe it is an option that must be tried, at least for a while. Likewise, a minority of individuals indicates that supplements also must be tried despite no proven effectiveness. Overall, family members say whether or not drugs or supplements worked was less important than knowing that everything possible was being tried.

Q: *What types of help have been most effective in planning for the future or making decisions?*

Apart from help provided by other family members and friends, most people report seeking out services to help in planning for the future. Most people note that getting legal and financial affairs in order is a top priority and, therefore, they had consulted a local elder law attorney. They also report getting good information about AD and other resources at local chapters of the Alzheimer's Association or the Alzheimer Society. A number of computer-savvy individuals say they looked to the Internet for information and found websites and bulletin boards to be useful.

Many people say that they eventually sought out support groups and found good opportunities for information and camaraderie with others dealing with similar situations. These groups were described as vitally important in some cases. One wife says that the people in the support group give her confidence that she can face the future, "It's like being pregnant for the first time. I was petrified and thought I would not survive it. Then I thought of all those women through the ages that had survived perfectly well so surely I would." A husband describes a deep attachment to a men's support group and says he drives 170 miles twice a month to participate. A few family members note that information shared in support groups is not always reliable or consistent. Some people tell of dropping out of support groups after awhile or never taking part in them at all. A few say that individual counseling on a private basis was a worthwhile investment.

Several older spouses say that the best preparation for their future involved choosing a continuing care retirement community. With several levels of care and a staff of professionals, this setting affords them permanent security as well as daily opportunities for socialization with other older adults. Moreover, they say that not having to rely on their adult children all of the time is a great relief.

Q: *What has been the most challenging aspect of dealing with the disease thus far?*

Responses to this question vary from person to person. Some people focus on daily care issues such as household and personal care tasks or engaging a loved one with activities. Juggling all of these responsibilities is truly stressful in such cases. However, most people consider the emotional aspects to be most challenging. For example, overcoming denial and reaching acceptance of mental decline by a spouse or parent was seen as critical. One woman refers to the first few years of her husband's AD as "the turmoil period." A daughter-in-law notes that, "Getting everyone in the family on the same page has been a cause of many heated disagreements. People clearly move at a different pace accepting the reality of Alzheimer's. The challenge is to make sure that everyone is kept well informed since emotions can get out of hand if [all family members are] not kept in the loop."

Many people describe a fine line between trying to keep the relationship as normal as possible and taking into account the changes in a loved one due to AD. A wife notes, "It's been difficult to continue participating in activities such as golf, bowling, gardening, and socializing with friends. You have to change gears often and figure out new ways to make these things continue smoothly. Sometimes you have to stop altogether." Many people describe difficulty getting other relatives and friends to understand what is happening and how to be involved. A husband says, "I needed to be specific about what I wanted from others, or otherwise, they would not know. At first, I guess I expected them to read my mind. It has gotten better now that they have some direct experience of caring for my wife."

Q: *What has been most useful in dealing with day-to-day care issues?*

If relatives and friends were available, their help was considered most useful. However, most people eventually tell of seeking out additional resources such as a paid helper or an adult day center. Anything done at home or at a day center to keep the person with AD positively engaged with activities or people is seen as useful. Several individuals tell of the critical role of adult day centers in giving them relief from care responsibilities and helping their relatives with AD enjoy time away from home. In addition, they say that staff members of day centers offer a wealth of information and support. A wife notes, "The women who run the day center are my angels. They have helped me keep my sanity while keeping my husband happy."

Several individuals warn about "not doing this alone" and the need to get relief for one's own welfare. A man came to the following realization in relation to his wife with AD: "When she is having a bad day, and I'm having a good day, life is manageable. When she is having a good day, and I'm having a bad day, life is manageable, too. When both of you are having bad days, then you need help." A son reports, "Once I got solid professional help, I could take charge and be proactive for a change." A wife notes, "I felt guilty at first for doing enjoyable things apart from him. I eventually learned that although he preferred me at all times, others could substitute. I would come back home feeling refreshed." A daughter notes that her mother was resistant to any form of help until an older woman was introduced as a "friend," secretly paid by the daughter.

Q: *What have you found most useful in coping with your emotions over the course of the disease?*

Most people found a number of coping strategies to be useful. Most individuals describe feelings of loss and difficulty accepting changes in their relationship with the person with AD. A wife reports that her greatest difficulty was in being honest about her feelings, "especially the dark ones." Self-relaxation techniques, prayer, physical exercise, support groups, and humor were among the most commonly used ways of coping with difficult emotions. Talking with a friend or a counselor was also useful for a number of people, especially spouses. A husband notes, "Until I was able to step outside of our relationship and deal with it almost in the third person, I had a lot of sad days." For adult children who are married, having a supportive spouse is seen as invaluable to work through difficult emotions. Those who are employed often look to their jobs as a good outlet.

Many individuals write of discovering a sense of satisfaction and meaning in the current situation. This typically grows out of crisis that is resolved by reframing or renegotiating their relationship with the person with AD. A husband writes, "After I got through my deep anger, I found out how to love my wife in profoundly simple ways." A daughter says, "When I stopped looking to my dad to control himself and focused instead on understanding him, I was better able to handle my emotions." One woman looks upon her husband's AD as "a project" that she is determined to cope with successfully on a day-to-day basis. A man who practices Buddhist meditation refers to his wife's disease as the "Alzheimer's opportunity" in which both he and his wife can be transformed into their essential selves.

Q: *What are you most hopeful about? Even if a cure or a treatment to stop Alzheimer's is not found soon, what keeps you going?*

Relatively few people cling to the hope for a cure or better medical treatments. The vast majority expresses the realization that scientific advances will not be available in time for their benefit. While generally hopeful that future generations will benefit from biomedical research, they now focus their attention on coping with everyday concerns of the caring relationship. Hope for today seems to be enough in most cases. A husband writes, "I have no hope for a medical breakthrough, but what keeps me going is the love I have for my wife." A wife notes, "I think a cure will be found some day but too late for us. Meanwhile, taking one day at a time seems to work best. Every new today is mine."

A daughter's goal is put simply: "I just want my dad to finish well, and I am most hopeful that I can make this happen." A husband declares, "I just want to outlive my wife and see that she gets the best possible care." A wife echoes this sentiment: "I just hope that I can remain healthy and strong and see my husband right through to the end." Another wife expresses her view succinctly: "I see no hope for a cure. What keeps me going is love, pure and simple."

Others have a more philosophical outlook. A wife remarks, "I am most hopeful for a cure for our children and grandchildren. In the meantime, what keeps me going is the belief that there is a plan for my life. I accept the hand I've been dealt." A son says, "What keeps me going is the certainty that I am always learning from other people and experience. Change is possible to fit any situation." A daughter adds, "I don't look for a cure or better medical treatment. I look for ways to rekindle the spirit—both hers and mine." A husband says, "I have no illusions about a miracle cure. I am most hopeful that I can look ahead now instead of looking back. This adjustment in my attitude is what enables me to take care of my wife." A son says, "I am not necessarily hopeful for a cure but for a better understanding that we can enjoy the moment and be better able to offer dignity and quality of life to older people." A daughter-in-law says, "I am hopeful that future generations won't have to face Alzheimer's. My faith keeps me going for now."

Q: *What has been the best part, if any, of caring for someone with Alzheimer's disease? In other words, has anything good come out of this experience for you?*

This question evoked perhaps the most interesting responses. A few people chose not to respond at all and another small minority indicated that the negatives outweighed the positives. For example, a wife writes, "I do not see any good coming from what I see as a slow death. But I know he would do the same for me if roles were reversed." Another wife observes, "To be honest, I don't see anything positive about this. I guess it's good that I am coping and that my husband is happy. And there will be life after Alzheimer's." A wife writes, "So far nothing but frustration has come from my husband's Alzheimer's. He's easy to talk to, but he forgets everything."

However, most people write about the surprising benefits of caring for someone with AD. This experience often had resulted in an improved relationship with the person with AD or other family members and friends. Above all, this experience brought forth a personal resiliency and intense resolve that would have been unimaginable previously. The following quotes attest to the transforming nature of the care experience:

> I am a better person now, more patient and tolerant, less self-centered. I am glad to help my husband who has always helped me.

> Once I got in touch with my unconditional love, I took care of my wife because I wanted to and not because I had to. It has deepened my spiritual life and made me more aware of other's suffering. I have become more socially responsible.

> From being part of a support group, I have learned much about devotion and loving kindness. I am grateful for the chance to meet such amazing people. They are unsung heroes and heroines.

> The best part of this is knowing that our love still endures.

> He relies on me for everything, and sometimes I feel smothered. Yet we have grown closer. I continue to grow stronger every day on my own, too. I now do things that I never dreamed possible.

> Alzheimer's has lifted mother's inhibitions. Although a cause for embarrassment at times, she is now a far more happy and lovable person than in the past. I feel so blessed to have this time with her.

> Now, instead of fighting what fate has put before me, I can see in hindsight that I have been enriched by this experience. While cynics may think this makes me sound like Pollyanna, there have been points along this frequently dark road where I have felt blessed and rewarded. I am also satisfied knowing that I have made a

positive difference in my mother-in-law's quality of life. I know she appreciates the effort, too.

I have come to love my mother very deeply and to appreciate [that] her essence as a person remains and responds to love, care, humor, joy, and closeness. I have come to understand a deeper form of intimacy beyond words.

I have more fun with my dad now than I ever have. He was always doing guy stuff when I was growing up, but now he's there for me to talk with about the past and laugh. I could not wire circuits with him before, but now we enjoy separating Legos by color. Go figure…a blessing in the midst of this!

Caring for my husband has enlightened me to the depth and expanse of the strength and patience I possess, much more than I was ever aware of before being faced with this challenge. We both had the joy of family, friends, and neighbors who have been with us on this journey.

I have put aside the things that separated me from my mother—so much stuff that doesn't really matter. I have also been able to get along better with my siblings.

I have learned patience, how to listen and empathize. But it is a heck of a way to learn. I have never known so much pain.

Although I am still trying to overcome my anger and frustration, I see that we have grown closer together as a family.

My dad's disease has advanced to the degree that he no longer recognizes me, but I am grateful that he feels loved. The best part is knowing that he is truly happy in spite of Alzheimer's.

It would be better if my father did not have this disease, but the best thing I have found out is that my husband is a wonderful and caring son-in-law.

We are now closer as an entire family as we work together to care for my mother-in-law. Also, my mother-in-law is less guarded and [more] accepting of our assistance. She is more appreciative and pleasant than in the past.

I have learned to treasure the memories of all the good years instead of mourning the loss of the years we might have had together.

A social worker who had worked with individuals and families affected by AD prior to the onset of her own mother's AD reports:

> Having this personal experience both deepened and added another dimension to my professional life. I don't mean to say that professionals who don't have this experience can't be excellent— there are many. Another positive is the loving, intimate, and spiritual connection it provided both my mother and me. We would not have reached this level in our relationship without her Alzheimer's. It was truly a gift.

Lessons Learned

It is difficult to encapsulate the varied experiences of people who have cared for a loved one with AD. It is even more difficult to explain why people cope poorly or well with a similar set of challenges day after day, year after year. The quality of one's past relationship with the person with AD undoubtedly influences one's coping ability. The amount and frequency of social supports certainly make a difference, too. Other personal resources such as time and money can also play roles. A vast amount of social research in recent years has looked at a variety of factors that help explain why some people cope poorly and why others cope well caring for someone with AD. An interesting finding has emerged: Above all else, how one perceives the situation accounts for much of the difference in whether one copes poorly or well.

Those who see this situation as an ongoing tragedy typically respond to the stressors with depression, anxiety, and a host of other problems. They perceive no positive results from their hard work, and they often feel depleted. The deterioration of a loved one's mind is a cause for daily sadness. They see little or nothing good in the present situation and truly suffer through an endless funeral. Despair is an everyday reality, and the future looks grim.

On the other hand, those people who learn to see AD as an opportunity to achieve personal meaning, mission, or purpose are likely to cope well. Their countless acts of devotion, although draining at times, lead them not to despair but to confirmation that each day is worthwhile. They accept the limits imposed by the disease yet try to realize the potential in every encounter and act of care. They see problems as challenges that can lead to personal growth. They see with eyes of faith, irrespective of a religious bent, and understand that a broken mind or body is not the ultimate tragedy. They are most concerned with care of the soul—their loved one's and their own.

You cannot give what you do not have. If you cannot be open to the possibilities presented by AD, then seek out help—you will be amazed to find other people who have learned to thrive, not just survive. You can change your attitude and behavior to adapt to this life-changing situation. Human resilience in the face of adversity is a wonder to behold. The person with AD will ultimately benefit from your personal struggle, and you will eventually grow into a better person. This may seem unimaginable right now, but it can happen.

Finally, I wish to end with a call for courage. You have an awesome responsibility to ensure that someone with AD lives life to the fullest, no matter how radically that may differ from his or her past standards. At the same time, you also must make sure that your life is kept in balance in spite of the sacrifices you make every day. Winston Churchill implored the people of Great Britain in the darkest hours of World War II to continue struggling for hope. His inspiring message may well apply to you now:

"Never give in, never give in, never, never, never, never—in nothing, great or small, large or petty—never give in except to convictions of honor and good sense."

Epilogue:
Advocating for Change

*It is not enough for a great nation merely
to have added new years to life. Our objective
must also be to add new life to those years.*
President John F. Kennedy

If you are a relative or friend directly involved in providing care to someone with AD, you spend a lot of time and energy dealing with it every day. Although the problems associated with the disease are shared by millions of people, your focus is probably not on the larger social context. Your concerns for now are personal and rightly so. At present, it may be unrealistic for you to be involved in advocating for changes in public policy that would improve care and lead to better treatments or prevention. However, you should be aware of the larger issues in the political arena. The problem of AD is far too big and complex for any individual or family to solve, and advocates are needed in long-running battles over public policy and funding.

Until recent generations, most people lived in close proximity to their extended families. Mutual assistance in caring for the needs of the young and the old alike was a clear expectation in society. Responsibility of caring for a sick or disabled relative was shared among members of the family. For a variety of reasons, families ordinarily do not enjoy such close ties today, and members may live long distances from each other. The responsibility of caring for the younger and older generations is now shared by fewer family members than ever before in human history. Too often the care of someone with a chronic illness like AD falls on the shoulders of one person. No individual can successfully meet the complex needs of someone with the disease. Various forms of help, such as that provided by relatives, employers, neighbors, friends, churches, civic organizations, and government programs are needed.

Hillary Rodham Clinton once wrote a book about social responsibility based on the African adage "It takes a village to raise a child." She was unfairly criticized for allegedly trying to substitute government for the role of individuals. She responded by saying that the task of child rearing is so crucial to society that it needs to be seen as both a personal and collective obligation. This same argument might well apply to the task of caring for someone with AD. The disease takes a heavy toll on society—everyone pays, either directly or indirectly. And AD presents enormous financial problems as well, costing more than $200 billion annually in the United States alone in payments for health care, long-term care, and hospice, mostly through Medicare and Medicaid. And the economic value of unpaid care provided by family and friends is estimated to be more than $200 billion annually.[1] These huge costs will continue to escalate as the number of people with AD increases in the coming decades.

The Politics of Health Care

Any time huge numbers of Americans have been affected by a health problem as significant as AD, a political movement has taken shape to demand more funding for research and improved care. The public health problems of tuberculosis and polio in past generations led to massive increases in government expenditure to deal with these illnesses. More recently, significant increases in government spending for AIDS and breast cancer research can be traced to advocacy by people with these diseases, their loved ones, and health-care professionals. The AIDS crisis in particular, which began in the early 1980s, focused the public's attention like no other health problem had in recent times. Advocacy efforts clearly paid off as shown by breakthroughs in treating and preventing AIDS. The organized efforts of advocates can clearly instill the political will to increase government funding for care, treatment, and prevention of diseases.

The problem of AD does not yet have a high profile in spite of the staggering human and financial costs. Those with the disease are seldom able to speak for themselves. They cannot mount letter-writing campaigns, march in public demonstrations, or lobby elected officials to express dissatisfaction over the state of funding for care, treatment, and prevention. For the most part, they are older people who are hidden in the shadows and easily ignored by the rest of society. They are often considered "over the hill" and hold no political power. Furthermore, their loved ones, directly engaged in caring for them, are often too busy to be involved in a political movement.

The Alzheimer's Association, the Alzheimer Society, and similar organizations have been remarkably effective in increasing public awareness and raising federal allocations for AD research every year over the past thirty years. And increasing numbers of people in the early stages of the disease have joined this effort. Although the total amount allocated for AD research from U.S. government funds continues to grow each year, research expenditures pale in comparison to other major public health problems. The effort needs advocates to raise funds and to pressure every single elected official to allocate a much bigger portion of government funds. I urge you to get involved with advocacy organizations as time allows for this important work. In the meantime, encourage your circle of relatives and friends to champion this cause.

If concern about the health of our elders does not generate public concern about AD, then self-interest should. By the year 2050, as many as fourteen million Americans and more than a hundred million people worldwide will have the disease. Women in particular carry a greater burden than men in relation to AD. Not only do more women than men have AD, but women provide a disproportionate amount of care to people with the disease. The disease should be championed as a women's health issue akin to breast cancer.

It does not take a crystal ball to predict what will happen in the decades ahead. This costly disease will affect huge numbers of people—those who need care, those who provide care, and everyone else who will pay for that care in one way or another. It is as if we are standing at the ocean's shore and can see a tsunami approaching, all the while hoping that science will solve the problem before the waves hit home. Wishful thinking will not make the problem go away. Action must be taken now.

The Role of Government

Progress is being made to find better treatments and means of prevention for AD. Preventing the disease is the ultimate goal of biomedical research, yet this is still just a dream. The late Dr. Robert Butler, former director of the National Institute on Aging, once cautioned:

> We remain ill-prepared for the twenty-first century when population aging will become unprecedented. I regard the baby boomers as a generation at risk. We still devote relatively few resources to understanding the biology of aging. Although we have made progress in understanding the pathogenesis of Alzheimer's disease, we are a long way from a cure.

Despite significant advances over the past two decades, it may take many more decades before dramatic results can be seen. Scientific efforts need better funding to speed up the rate of progress. This is the impetus behind the National Alzheimer's Project Act, signed into law in 2011, which requires an annually updated National Plan to Address Alzheimer's Disease.[2] Thus far, an Advisory Council on Alzheimer's Research, Care, and Services has established four main goals:

1. prevent and effectively treat AD by 2025
2. optimize care quality and efficiency
3. expand supports for people with AD and families
4. enhance public awareness and engagement

To achieve these goals, it is estimated that $2 billion dollars is needed annually, more than four times the amount currently spent by the U.S. government for AD medical research. This increase would begin to put the disease on a par with cancer, heart disease, diabetes, and AIDS. Devoting just a fraction of that amount to find better ways of caring for people with the disease through nonmedical means would highlight that enhancing quality of life is a legitimate goal of care.

The fate of millions of people affected by the disease cannot be shouldered entirely by the hard-working scientists aiming to unlock the mysteries of AD. We—our society and government—must give increased attention to helping those people who are currently coping with the disease and may never taste the fruits of scientific advances. Their quality of life now depends more on human compassion and skill than on new medical breakthroughs. What can be done to help individuals and families on a practical level? Here are just a few ideas:

- At all levels of government, we must find better alternatives to nursing-home care, such as home care, assisted-living facilities, and other supportive living arrangements.

- Families need easy access to affordable respite care and other services to support them in their role as the main providers of care. A comprehensive family support network must be established. In the United States, the National Family Caregiving Support Program is making a positive difference, but this program needs a big budget boost.

- Family members and others who provide direct care should receive increased tax credits in recognition of their hard work and cost savings to society.

- Families need free access to Web-based training programs about coping with AD.

The Role of the Private Sector

Government alone cannot solve the range of problems associated with AD. Business already pays a high price for this disease, at least $75 billion annually, according to a survey commissioned by the Alzheimer's Association.[3] It is estimated that absenteeism and tardiness affect one-third of employees who care for relatives with AD, and 10 percent of these people quit their jobs each year because of their competing roles at work and at home. In response to such family-related concerns, many employers have developed family-assistance programs. These include benefits such as:

- unpaid leave beyond the twelve-week leave required by the U.S. Family and Medical Leave Act that also guarantees workers retention of full medical and dental benefits, enabling workers to use their sick leave to care for a disabled relative

- referral services linking employees to services nationwide, making it possible to arrange care for a relative who lives either locally or far away

- reimbursement for services paid for a disabled relative, similar to child-care reimbursement

- long-term-care insurance packages for employees, spouses, parents, and in-laws

- counseling for employees and their families affected by care responsibilities

Government agencies, businesses, and nonprofit organizations working together can have powerful effects on the quality of life for individuals and families affected by AD. For example, AmeriCorps, a national service program of the U.S. government that subsidizes volunteers working with nonprofits, could make AD a priority area and focus on services to people affected by the disease. Philanthropic organizations, too, could adopt AD as their central focus. Rotary International, for example, has nearly succeeded in eliminating the worldwide scourge of polio after decades of hard work. Similar organizations could make a long-term commitment with respect to AD. An army of volunteers from churches and schools might tackle the worldwide problem of AD. The monthly "Alzheimer's Cafes" springing up in Europe, Canada, and the United States illustrate how private organizations can bring together people with AD, their families, volunteers, and professionals for education and support in a social setting.

The relatively brief history of research into the causes, treatment, and prevention of AD has had many ups and downs. Certainly, far more experimental drugs have failed than proven effective. Success in the end will depend in large part on funding from public and private sources. The goal of preventing AD has a chance of being achieved when a critical mass of people decides that this is a priority worth funding on a grand scale. In the meantime, the goal of improving the quality of life of millions of individuals and families affected by the disease requires more money, too.

Reaching these lofty goals will take a massive collective effort. The sign that President Ronald Reagan kept on his desk in the Oval Office might well be adopted as the motto of everyone involved in this undertaking: IT CAN BE DONE. This same sense of optimism must fuel the hopes of all who are concerned about this mind-robbing disease, especially those living with the disease who can no longer speak for themselves.

Notes

Chapter 1: The Need for an Accurate Diagnosis

1. N. D. Anderson, K. J. Murphy, and A. K. Troyer, *Living with Mild Cognitive Impairment: A Guide to Maximizing Brain Health and Reducing Risk of Dementia* (New York: Oxford University Press, 2012).

2. M. S. Albert et al., "The Diagnosis of Mild Cognitive Impairment Due to Alzheimer's Disease: Recommendations from the National Institute on Aging-Alzheimer's Association Workgroups on Diagnostic Guidelines for Alzheimer's Disease," *Alzheimer's & Dementia: The Journal of the Alzheimer's Association* 7, no. 3 (2011): 270–79; G. M. McKhann et al., "The Diagnosis of Dementia Due to Alzheimer's Disease: Recommendations from the National Institute on Aging-Alzheimer's Association Workgroups on Diagnostic Guidelines for Alzheimer's Disease," *Alzheimer's & Dementia: The Journal of the Alzheimer's Association* 7, no. 3 (2011): 263–69; New Diagnostic Criteria and Guidelines for Alzheimer's Disease, 2011, http://www.alz.org/research/diagnostic_criteria. (accessed 26 May 2013).

3. Ibid.

4. Ibid.

5. K. L. Howard and C. M. Filley, "Advances in Genetic Testing for Alzheimer's Disease," *Reviews in Neurological Diseases* 6, no. 1 (2009): 26–32.

6. J. S. Goldman et al., "Genetic Counseling and Testing for Alzheimer Disease: Joint Practice Guidelines of the American College of Medical Genetics and the National Society of Genetic Counselors," *Genetic Medicine* 13, no. 6 (2011): 597–605.

7. K. Maurer, S. Volk, and H. Gerbaldo, "Auguste D. amd Alzheimer's Disease," *The Lancet* 349 (1997): 1546–49; K. Maurer and U. Maurer, *Alzheimer: The Life of a Physician & the Career of a Disease* (New York: Columbia University Press, 2003).

8. U. Muller, P. Winter, and M, B. Graeber, "A Presenilin Mutation in the First Case of Alzheimer's Disease," *The Lancet Neurology* 12, no. 2 (2013): 129–30.

9. L. Hebert et al., "Alzheimer Disease in the United States (2010–2050) Estimated Using the 2010 Census," *Neurology* 13, no. 6 (2013): 1778–83.

10. L. Radin and G. Radin, *What If It's Not Alzheimer's? A Caregiver's Guide to Dementia* (Amherst, NY: Prometheus Books, 2008).

11. M. F. Folstein, S. E. Folstein, and P. R. McHugh, "Mini-Mental State: A Practical Method for Grading the Cognitive State of Patients for the Clinician," *Journal of Psychiatric Research* 12 (1975): 189–98.

12. S. Borson et al., "Mini-Cog: A Cognitive 'Vital Signs' Measure for Dementia Screening in Multi-Lingual Elderly," *International Journal of Geriatric Psychiatry* 15, no. 11 (2000): 1021–27.

13. Alzheimer's Association, *Principles for a Dignified Diagnosis* (Chicago, IL: Alzheimer's Association, 2009), http://www.alz.org/national /documents/brochure_dignified_diagnosis.pdf (accessed 26 May 2013).

Chapter 2: Symptoms of the Early Stages of Alzheimer's Disease

1. R. Reagan, "Open Letter to the American Public" (4 November 1994).

2. M. J. Zuckerman, "Bush: Reagan Wasn't Ill as President," *USA Today*, 29 November 1996.

3. E. Morris, *Dutch: A Memoir of Ronald Reagan* (New York: Random House, 1999).

4. A. Davidson, *Alzheimer's, A Love Story: One Year in My Husband's Journey* (Secaucus, NJ: Carol Publishing Group, 1997), 184.

5. A. Bradford et al., "Missed and Delayed Diagnosis of Dementia in Primary Care: Prevalence and Contributing Factors," *Alzheimer's Disease and Associated Disorders* 23, no. 4 (2009): 306–14.

6. S. Weintraub, A. H. Wicklund, and D. P. Salmon, "The Neuropsychological Profile of Alzheimer's Disease," *Cold Spring Harbor Perspectives in Medicine* 2, no. 4 (2012).

7. H. R. Sohrabi et al., "Olfactory Discrimination Predicts Cognitive Decline among Community-Dwelling Older Adults," *Translational Psychiatry* 2, no. 5 (2012).

8. C. B. Cordell et al., "Alzheimer's Association Recommendations for Operationalizing the Detection of Cognitive Impairment During the Medicare Annual Wellness Visit in a Primary Care Setting," *Alzheimer's & Dementia: The Journal of the Alzheimer's Association* 9, no. 2 (2013).

Chapter 3: Treatment and Prevention of Alzheimer's Disease

1. S.Birks, "Cholinesterase Inhibitors for Alzheimer's Disease." Cochrane

Database for Systematic Reviews 25, no. 1, (25 January 2006): CD005593.

2. S. A. Areosa, F. Sherriff, and R. McShane, "Memantine for Dementia," *Cochrane Database for Systematic Reviews* no. 2 (19 April 2006): CD003154.

3. T. Muayquil and R. Camicioli, "Systematic Review and Meta-Analysis of Combination Therapy with Cholinesterase Inhibitors and Memantine in Alzheimer's Disease and Other Dementias," *Dementia & Geriatric Cognitive Disorders* 2, no. 1 (2012): 546–72.

4. S. T. Henderson et al., "Study of the Ketogenic Agent AC-1202 in Mild to Moderate Alzheimer's Disease: A Randomized, Double-Blind, Placebo-Controlled, Multicenter Trial," *Nutrition & Metabolism* 6, no. 31 (2009).

5. P. Scheltens et al., "Efficacy of Soubenaid in Mild Alzheimers's Disease: Results from a Randomized, Controlled Trial," *Journal of Alzheimer's Disease* 31, no. 1 (2012): 225–36.

6. S. DeKosky et al., "Ginkgo Biloba for Prevention of Dementia: A Randomized Controlled Trial," *Journal of the American Medical Association* 300, no. 19 (2008): 2253–62; B. Vellas et al., "Long-Term Use of Standardised Ginkgo Biloba Extract for the Prevention of Alzheimer's Disease (GuidAge): A Randomised Placebo-Controlled Trial," *Lancet Neurology* 11, no. 10 (2012): 851–59.

7. Rafii et al., "A Phase II Trial of Huperzine A in Mild to Moderate Alzheimer Disease," *Neurology* 76, no. 16 (2011): 1389–94; J. Li et al., "Huperzine A for Alzheimer's Disease," *Cochrane Database for Systematic Reviews* no. 2 (16 Apr 2008): CD005592.

8. N. T. Lautenschlager et al., "Effect of Physical Activity on Cognitive Function in Older Adults at Risk for Alzheimer Disease: A Randomized Trial," *Journal of the American Medical Association* 300, no. 9 (2008): 1027–37; R. S. Wilson et al., "Participation in Cognitively Stimulating Activities and Risk of Incident Alzheimer Disease," *Journal of the American Medical Association* 287, no. 6 (2002): 742–48.

9. National Institutes of Health, *Preventing Alzheimer's Disease and Cognitive Decline*, The Report of the National Institutes of Health State -of-the-Science Conference, April 26–28, 2010, http://consensus.nih .gov/2010/alz.htm (accessed 28 May 2013).

10. Alzheimer's Research Forum, "NIH Director Announces $100M Prevention Trial of Genentech Antibody," http://www.alzforum.org/new

/detail.asp?id=3155 (accessed 24 May 2013); National Institutes of Health, "NIH-Supported Alzheimer's Studies to Focus on Innovative Treatment," http://www.nih.gov/news/health/jan2013/nia-14.htm (accessed 24 May 2013).

11. Quoted in W. B. Bean, *Sir William Osler: Aphorisms from His Bedside Teachings and Writings* (Springfield, IL: Charles C. Thomas, 1961), 77.

12. R. Taylor, *Alzheimer's from the Inside Out* (Baltimore, MD: Health Professions Press, 2006), 112.

Chapter 4: A Good Quality of Life

1. O. Ames Hoblitzelle, *Ten Thousand Joys and Ten Thousand Sorrows: A Couple's Journey Through Alzheimer's* (New York: Tarcher, 2010), 5.

2. G. A. Power, *Dementia Beyond Drugs: Changing the Culture of Care* (Baltimore, MD: Health Professions Press, 2010).

3. T. Kitwood, *Dementia Reconsidered: The Person Comes First* (Buckingham, England: Open University Press, 1997).

4. E. Voris, N. Shabahangi, and P. Fox, *Conversations with Ed: Waiting for Forgetfulness: Why Are We So Afraid of Alzheimer's Disease?* (San Francisco, CA: Elders Academy Press, 2009).

Chapter 5: What Is It Like to Have Alzheimer's Disease?

1. L. Genova, *Still Alice* (New York: Gallery Books, 2009).

2. C. Henderson et al., *Partial View: An Alzheimer's Journal* (Dallas, TX: Southern Methodist University Press, 1998), 36.

3. Henderson, *Partial View*, 55.

4. R. Davis, *My Journey into Alzheimer's Disease* (Wheaton, IL: Tyndale House Publishers, 1989), 100.

5. L. Rose, *Show Me the Way to Go Home* (Forest Knolls, CA: Elder Books, 1996), 35.

6. C. Boden, *Who Will I Be When I Die?* (East Melbourne, Australia: HarperCollins Religious, 1998), 53.

7. Davis, *My Journey into Alzheimer's Disease*, 107.

8. Henderson, *Partial View*, 36.

9. D. Friel McGowin, *Living in the Labyrinth: A Personal Journey Through the Maze of Alzheimer's* (New York: Delacorte Press, 1993), 8.

10. Davis, *My Journey into Alzheimer's Disease*, 107.

11. Boden, *Who Will I Be When I Die?*, 49.

12. Rose, *Show Me the Way to Go Home*, 126.

13. McGowin, *Living in the Labyrinth*, 87.

14. T. M. Raushi, *A View from Within: Living with Early Onset Alzheimer's* (Albany, NY: Northeastern Chapter of the Alzheimer's Association, 2001), 119.

15. R. Reagan, "Open Letter to the American Public," (4 November 1994).

16. S. G. Post, *The Moral Challenge of Alzheimer's Disease* (Baltimore, MD: The Johns Hopkins University Press, 1995), 15.

17. C. Heston, "Open Letter to Friends, Colleagues and Fans," (9 August 2002).

18. R. Taylor, *Alzheimer's from the Inside Out* (Baltimore, MD: Health Professions Press, 2006), 78.

19. D. Baron, "Alzheimer's Disease: Living with It," *Chicago Sun-Times*, 2 November 1992, 3A, 15.

20. K. Maurer, S.Volk, and H. Gerbaldo, "Auguste D and Alzheimer's Disease," *The Lancet* 349 (1997): 1546–49.

21. Boden, *Who Will I Be When I Die?*, 145.

Chapter 6: How Relationships, Roles, and Responsibilities Change

1. C. M. Clark, *Caring About Howard: Alzheimer's Disease as a Shared Journey* (Durham, NC: Educational Media Services in association with Lisa Gwyther, Duke University Medical Center, 1997), video.

2. P. H. Summitt and S. Jenkins, *Sum It Up: A Thousand and Ninety-Eight Victories, a Couple of Irrelevant Losses, and a Life in Perspective* (New York: Crown Archetype, 2013), 132.

3. W. Lustbader, *Counting on Kindness: The Dilemmas of Dependency* (New York: The Free Press, 1992), 79.

4. M. L'Engle, *The Summer of the Great-Grandmother* (New York: Farrar, Strauss & Giroux, 1974), 187.

5. Educational Media Services and L. P. Gwyther, *From Here to Hope: The Stages of Alzheimer's Disease* (Durham, NC: Duke University Medical Center, 1998), video.

6. M. Shriver, *What's Happening to Grandpa?* (New York: Little, Brown Books for Young Readers, 2004).

7. Alzheimer's Association, *Alzheimer's Disease: Inside Looking Out* (Cleveland, OH: Cleveland Area Chapter, 1995), video.

8. C. Boden, *Who Will I Be When I Die?* (East Melbourne, Australia: HarperCollins Religious, 1998), 58.

Chapter 7: Making Practical Decisions

1. M. Man-Son-Hing et al., "Systematic Review of Driving Risk and the

Efficacy of Compensatory Strategies in Persons with Dementia," *Journal of the American Geriatrics Society* 55, no. 6 (2007): 878–84.

2. HBO Films, *The Memory Loss Tapes*, video. One of four documentaries produced in 2009 for the series, *The Alzheimer's Project*. Can be viewed for free at: www.hbo.com/alzheimers.

3. P. A. Webber, P. Fox, and D. Burnette, "Living Alone with Alzheimer's Disease: Effects on Health and Social Service Utilization Patterns," *The Gerontologist* 34, no. 1 (1994): 8–14.

4. B. B. Murphy, *He Used to Be Somebody: A Journey into Alzheimer's Disease Through the Eyes of a Caregiver* (Boulder, CO: Gibbs Associates, 1995), 311.

Chapter 8: Improving Communication

1. T. Kitwood, *Dementia Reconsidered: The Person Comes First* (Buckingham, England: Open University Press, 1997), 57.

2. R. Davis, *My Journey into Alzheimer's Disease* (Wheaton, IL: Tyndale House Publishers, 1989), 85–86.

3. T. Raushi, *A View from Within: Living with Early Onset Alzheimer's* (Albany, NY: Northeastern Chapter of the Alzheimer's Association, 2001), 26.

4. Davis, *My Journey into Alzheimer's Disease*, 88.

5. C. Boden, *Who Will I Be When I Die?* (East Melbourne, Australia: HarperCollins Religious, 1998), 90.

6. P. Davis, *Angels Don't Die: My Father's Gift of Faith* (New York: HarperCollins Publishers, 1995), 36.

7. D. Hoffman, *Complaints of a Dutiful Daughter* (New York: Women Make Movies, 1995), video.

8. M. S. Bourgeois, *Memory Books and Other Graphic Cuing Systems: Practical Communication and Memory Aids for Adults with Dementia* (Baltimore, MD: Health Professions Press, 2007).

9. A. Davidson, *Alzheimer's, A Love Story: One Year in My Husband's Journey* (Secaucus, NJ: Carol Publishing Group, 1997), 193.

Chapter 9: Helping a Person with Alzheimer's Disease Plan for the Future

1. U.S. Department of Labor, "Family and Medical Leave Act," http://www.dol.gov/whd/fmla (accessed 25 May 2013).

2. U.S. Department of the Treasury, Internal Revenue Service, *Publication 502: Medical and Dental Services,* http://www.irs.gov/pub/irs-pdf/p502.pdf (accessed 25 May 2013); U.S. Department of the Treasury,

Internal Revenue Service, *Publication 502: Child and Dependent Care Expenses,* http://www.irs.gov/pub/irs-pdf/p503.pdf (accessed 25 May 2013).

3. AARP, *Home Made Money: A Consumer's Guide to Reverse Mortgages,* 2006, http://assets.aarp.org/www.aarp.org_/articles/revmort/home MadeMoney.pdf.

4. L. White and B. Spencer, *Moving a Relative with Memory Loss: A Family Caregiver's Guide* (Santa Rosa, CA: Whisp Publications, 2006).

Chapter 10: Keeping a Person with Alzheimer's Disease Active

1. J. M. Zgola, *Doing Things: A Guide to Programming Activities for Persons with Alzheimer's Disease and Related Disorders.* (Baltimore, MD: The Johns Hopkins University Press, 1987).

2. M. E. Geist, *Measure of the Heart: Caring for a Parent with Alzheimer's* (New York: Springboard Press, 2008), 61.

3. L. P. Gwyther, *You Are One of Us: Successful Clergy/Church Connections to Alzheimer's Families* (Durham, NC: Duke University Medical Center, 1995).

Chapter 11: Self-Renewal for Family and Friends

1. M. Mitchell, *Dancing on Quicksand: A Gift of Friendship in the Age of Alzheimer's* (Boulder, CO: Johnson Books, 2002).

2. E. Kübler-Ross, *On Death and Dying* (New York: Macmillan, 1969).

3. P. Davis, *The Long Goodbye: Memories of My Father* (New York: Knopf Doubleday Publishing Group, 2005).

4. W. Ewing, *Tears in God's Bottle: Reflections on Alzheimer's Caregiving* (Tucson, AZ: WhiteStone Circle Press, 1999), 106.

5. O. Ames Hoblitzelle, *Ten Thousand Joys and Ten Thousand Sorrows: A Couple's Journey Through Alzheimer's* (New York: Tarcher, 2010), 58.

6. S. Fish, *Alzheimer's: Caring for Your Loved One, Caring for Yourself* (Batavia, IL: Lion Publishing Company, 1990), 171.

7. J. Tucker, "How to Change Surviving into Thriving," *Rush Alzheimer's Disease Center News* (Spring 1995), 4.

Chapter 12: Obtaining the Help You May Need

1. J. Vanden Bosch, *A Thousand Tomorrows: Intimacy, Sexuality, and Alzheimer's* (Chicago, IL: Terra Nova Films, 1994), video.

Chapter 13: Voices of Experience

1. Alzheimer's Association, *Principles for a Dignified Diagnosis* (Chicago, IL: Alzheimer's Association, 2009), http://www.alz.org/national/documents/brochure_dignified_diagnosis.pdf (accessed 26 May 2013).

Epilogue: Advocating for Change

1. Alzheimer's Association, *2013 Alzheimer's Disease Facts and Figures* (Chicago, IL: Alzheimer's Association, 2013), http://www.alz.org/downloads/facts_figures_2013.pdf (accessed 26 May 2013).

2. National Alzheimer's Project Act, http://aspe.hhs.gov/daltcp/napa (accessed 13 August 2013).

3. R. Koppel, *Alzheimer's Disease: The Costs to U.S. Businesses in 2002* (Chicago, IL: Alzheimer's Association, 2002).

Additional Resources

Print, Video, and Web Resources

Chapter 1: The Need for an Accurate Diagnosis

Alzheimer's Association. *Ten Early Signs and Symptoms of Alzheimer's.* http://www.alz.org/10signs.

California Council. *Guidelines for Alzheimer's Disease Management.* Sacramento, CA: California Workgroup on Guidelines for Alzheimer's Disease, 2008. http://caalz.org/learn/guidelines.

Chapter 2: Symptoms of the Early Stages of Alzheimer's Disease

HBO Films. *Momentum in Science,* a documentary on the state-of-the-science by twenty-five leading scientists from the four-part series, *The Alzheimer's Project,* 2009. Available to view for free at http://www.hbo.com/alzheimers.

D. Shenk, J. Mallis, and D. Hyde Pierce. *A Quick Look at Alzheimer's.* Five short animated films about the medical aspects of the disease available for purchase and free viewing at http://www.AboutAlz.org.

Chapter 3: Treatment and Prevention of Alzheimer's Disease

Alzheimer's Disease Cooperative Study. A consortium of research centers funded by the U.S. government to conduct innovative research studies. http://www.adcs.org.

Doraiswamy, P. M., and L. P. Gwyther. *The Alzheimer's Action Plan: The Experts' Guide to the Best Diagnosis and Treatment for Memory Problems.* New York: St. Martin's Press, 2008.

Chapter 4: A Good Quality of Life

Bell, V., and D. Troxel. *A Dignified Life: The Best Friends Approach to Alzheimer's Care.* Deerfield Beach, FL: HCIBooks.com, 2012.

Snyder, L., *Living Your Best with Early-Stage Alzheimer's: An Essential Guide.* North Branch, MN: Sunrise River Press, 2010.

Murray Alzheimer Research and Education Program, University of Waterloo, Canada. "Living with Dementia: Resources for Living Well." http://livingwithdementia.uwaterloo.ca.

Chapter 5: What Is It Like to Have Alzheimer's Disease?

HBO Films. *The Memory Loss Tapes,* a documentary from the four-part series, *The Alzheimer's Project,* 2009. Available to view for free at http://www.hbo.com/alzheimers.

Braudy Harris, P. (Ed.). *The Person with Alzheimer's Disease: Pathways to Understanding the Experience.* Baltimore, MD: The Johns Hopkins University Press, 2002.

Snyder, L. *Speaking Our Minds: What It's Like to Have Alzheimer's.* Baltimore, MD: Health Professions Press, 2009.

Chapter 6: How Relationships, Roles, and Responsibilities Change

Boss, P. *Loving Someone Who Has Dementia: How to Find Hope While Coping with Stress and Grief.* New York: Jossey-Bass, 2011.

McCurry, S. M. *When a Family Member Has Dementia: Steps to Becoming a Resilient Caregiver.* Westport, CT: Praeger Publishers, 2006.

Terra Nova Films. "VideoCaregiving: A Visual Education Center for Family Caregivers." Free videos available at http://www.videocaregiving.org.

Chapter 7: Making Practical Decisions

The Healing Project (Ed.), *Voices of Alzheimer's Disease.* New York: Lachance Publishing, 2007.

Bowlby Sifton, C. *Navigating the Alzheimer's Journey: A Compass for Caregiving.* Baltimore, MD: Health Professions Press, 2004.

Caregiver Action Network. http://caregiveraction.org.

Chapter 8: Improving Communication

Koenig Coste, J. *Learning to Speak Alzheimer's: A Groundbreaking Approach for Everyone Dealing with the Disease.* New York: Houghton Mifflin Harcourt, 2004.

de Klerk-Rubin, V. *Validation Techniques for Dementia Care: The Family Caregiver's Guide to Improving Communication.* Baltimore, MD: Health Professions Press, 2007.

Robinson, A. B. Spencer, and L. White. *Understanding Difficult Behaviors: Some Practical Suggestions for Coping with Alzheimer's Disease and Related Illnesses*. Ypsilanti, MI: Eastern Michigan University, 2007.

Chapter 9: Helping a Person with Alzheimer's Disease Plan for the Future

Gross, J. *A Bittersweet Season: Caring for Our Aging Parents—and Ourselves*. New York: Vintage Books, 2012.

James, V. E. *The Alzheimer's Advisor: A Caregiver's Guide to Dealing with the Tough Legal and Practical Issues*. New York: AMACOM, 2008.

Mittelman, M., and C. Epstein. *The Alzheimer's Health Care Handbook: How to Get the Best Medical Care for Your Relative with Alzheimer's Disease, in and out of the Hospital*. Cambridge, MA: Marlowe and Company, 2003.

Chapter 10: Keeping a Person with Alzheimer's Disease Active

Bell, V., D. Troxel, T. Cox, and R. Hamon. *The Best Friends Book of Alzheimer's Activities* (two volumes). Baltimore, MD: Health Professions Press, 2004 and 2007. Also check out http://www.bestfriendsapproach.com.

Brackey, J. *Creating Moments of Joy: A Journal for Caregivers*. West Lafayette, IN: Purdue University Press, 2007.

Chapter 11: Self-Renewal for Family and Friends

Boss, P. *Loving Someone Who Has Dementia: How to Find Hope While Coping with Stress and Grief*. Hoboken, NJ: Jossey-Bass, 2011.

Cleland, M., V. L. Schmall, M. Studervant, and L. Congleton. *The Caregiver Helpbook: Powerful Tools for Caregivers*. Portland, OR: Powerful Tools for Caregivers, 2006.

Witrogen McLeod, B. *Caregiving: The Spiritual Journey of Love, Loss, and Renewal*. New York: John Wiley and Sons, 2000.

Chapter 12: Obtaining the Help You May Need

Bornstein, R. F., and M. A. Languirand. *When Someone You Love Needs Nursing Home, Assisted Living, or In-Home Care*. New York: William Morrow, 2009.

Mace, N. L., and P. V. Rabins. *The 36-Hour Day: A Family Guide to Caring for People with Alzheimer Disease, Other Dementias, and Memory Loss in Later Life*. Baltimore, MD: The Johns Hopkins University Press, 2012.

Kuhn, D., and J. Verity. *The Art of Dementia Care*. Stamford, CT: Delmar Cengage Learning, 2007.

Chapter 13: Voices of Experience

Greenblatt, C. *Love, Loss, and Laughter: Seeing Alzheimer's Differently*. Guilford, CT: Lyons Press, 2010.

Nouwen, H. J. M. *A Spirituality of Caregiving*. Nashville, TN: Upper Room, 2011.

Murphey, C. *When Someone You Love Has Alzheimer's: Daily Encouragement*. Kansas City, MO: Beacon Hill Press, 2004.

Epilogue: Advocating for Change

National Alzheimer's Project Act: http://aspe.hhs.gov/daltcp/napa

Alzheimer's Association: www.alz.org/join_the_cause_advocacy.asp

Research Centers in the U.S.
Funded by the National Institute on Aging

Arizona

Arizona Alzheimer's Disease Center
c/o Banner Alzheimer's Institute
901 E. Willetta St., Phoenix AZ 85006
(602) 239-6500   www.azalz.org

California

University of California, Davis Medical Center
Alzheimer's Disease Center
4860 Y St., Ste. 3700
Sacramento CA 95817-4540
(916) 734-5496   http://alzheimer.ucdavis.edu

University of California, Irvine
Alzheimer's Disease Research Center
UCI Institute for Memory Impairments and Neurological Disorders
1100 Gottschalk Medical Plaza
Irvine CA 92697-4285
(949) 824-2382   www.alz.uci.edu

University of California, Los Angeles
Alzheimer's Disease Research Center
10911 Weyburn Ave., Ste. 200
Los Angeles CA 90095-7226
(310) 794-3665   www.EastonAD.ucla.edu

University of California, San Diego
Shiley-Marcos Alzheimer's Disease Research Center
8950 Villa La Jolla Dr., Ste. C129
La Jolla CA 92037
(858) 622-5800   http://adrc.ucsd.edu

University of California, San Francisco
UCSF Memory and Aging Center
Sandler Neurosciences Center
675 Nelson Rising Ln., Ste. 190
San Francisco CA 94143-1207
(415) 476-6880   http://memory.ucsf.edu

University of Southern California
Alzheimer's Disease Research Center
Memory and Aging Center
1510 San Pablo St., HCCII, Ste. 3000
Los Angeles CA 90033
(323) 442-7600   www.usc.edu/dept/gero/ADRC

Georgia

Emory University
Alzheimer's Disease Research Center
Wesley Woods Health Center, 3rd Fl.
1841 Clifton Rd., NE
Atlanta GA 30329
(404) 728-6950   www.med.emory.edu/ADC

Illinois

Northwestern University Feinberg School of Medicine
Cognitive Neurology and Alzheimer's Disease Center
675 N. St. Claire, Galter 20-100
Chicago IL 60611
(312) 695-9627   www.brain.northwestern.edu

Rush University Medical Center
Rush Alzheimer's Disease Center
600 South Paulina St., Ste. 1026
Chicago IL 60612
(312) 942-3333   www.rush.edu/radc

Indiana

Indiana University School of Medicine
Indiana Alzheimer Disease Center
Indiana University Health Neuroscience Center
Goodman Hall #4199
355 W. 16th St.
Indianapolis IN 46202-7176
(317) 963-7426   http://iadc.iupui.edu

Kansas

University of Kansas School of Medicine
KU Alzheimer's Disease Center
KU Clinical Research Center
4350 Shawnee Mission Dr.
Fairway KS 66205
(913) 588-0555   www.kualzheimer.org

Kentucky

University of Kentucky
Alzheimer's Disease Center
Sanders-Brown Center on Aging, Rm. 101
800 South Limestone St.
Lexington KY 40536-0230
(859) 323-6040   www.mc.uky.edu/coa

Maryland

The Johns Hopkins University
Alzheimer's Disease Research Center
558 Ross Research Bldg.
720 Rutland Ave.
Baltimore MD 21205-2196
(410) 502-5164   www.alzresearch.org

Massachusetts

Boston University
Alzheimer's Disease Center
Edith Nourse Rogers Memorial Veterans Hospital
200 Spring Rd.
Bedford MA 01730
(781) 687-3240   www.bu.edu/alzresearch

Massachusetts General Hospital/Harvard Medical School
Alzheimer's Disease Research Center
MGH Memory Disorders Unit
Wang Ambulatory Care Center
15 Parkman St., 8th Fl., Ste. 835
Boston MA 02114
(617) 724-6387   http://madrc.org

Minnesota

Mayo Clinic
Alzheimer's Disease Research Center
4111 Highway 52 North
Rochester MN 55901
(507) 284-1324
http://mayoresearch.mayo.edu/mayo/research/alzheimers_center

Missouri

Washington University School of Medicine
Alzheimer's Disease Research Center
4488 Forest Park Ave., Ste. 130
St. Louis MO 63108-2293
(314) 286-2881   http://alzheimer.wustl.edu

New York

Columbia University Medical Center
Taub Center for Research on Alzheimer's Disease and the Aging Brain
630 W. 168th St., P&S Box 16
New York NY 10032
(212) 305-2077   www.alzheimercenter.org

Mount Sinai School of Medicine
Mary Sano, PhD, Director
Alzheimer's Disease Research Center
One Gustave L. Levy Pl., Box 1230
New York NY 10029-6574
(212) 241-8329
www.mssm.edu/research/centers/alzheimers-disease-research-center

New York University Langone Medical Center
Comprehensive Center on Brain Aging
145 E. 32nd St., 2nd Fl.
New York NY 10016
(212) 263-3210   www.med.nyu.edu/adc

Oregon

Oregon Health and Science University
Layton Aging and Alzheimer's Disease Center
3181 SW Sam Jackson Park Rd., Mail Code CR 131
Portland OR 97239-3098
(503) 494-6695   www.ohsu.edu/research/alzheimers

Pennsylvania

University of Pennsylvania School of Medicine
Penn Memory Center
The Perelman Center for Advanced Medicine
2400 Civic Center Blvd., 2nd Fl., South Pavilion
Philadelphia PA 19104
(215) 662-7810   www.uphs.upenn.edu/ADC

University of Pittsburgh
Alzheimer's Disease Research Center
UPMC Montefiore, 4th Fl., Ste. 421
200 Lothrop St.
Pittsburgh PA 15213
(412) 692-2700   www.adrc.pitt.edu

Texas

University of Texas, Southwestern Medical Center
Alzheimer's Disease Research Center

5323 Harry Hines Blvd.
Dallas TX 75390-8869
(214) 648-9376
www.utsouthwestern.edu/education/medical-school/departments
/neurology/programs/alzheimers-disease-center

Washington

University of Washington
Alzheimer's Disease Research Center
Veterans Affairs Puget Sound Health System
1660 S. Columbian Way
Seattle WA 98108
(206) 764-2069   www.uwadrc.org

Wisconsin

University of Wisconsin
Wisconsin Alzheimer's Disease Research Center
UW Memory Assessment Clinic
2880 University Ave.
Madison WI 53705
(608) 263-7740   http://adrc.wisc.edu

Organizations Dedicated to
Alzheimer's and Related Dementias

Alzheimer's Disease

Alzheimer's Association
225 N. Michigan Ave., 17th Fl.
Chicago IL 60601-7633
(800) 272-3900   www.alz.org

Alzheimer Society of Canada
20 Eglinton Ave. W., 16th Fl.
Toronto, Ontario M4R 1K8
(416) 488-8772   www.alzheimer.ca

Alzheimer's Foundation of America
322 8th Ave., 7th Fl.
New York NY 10001
(866) 232-8484   www.alzfdn.org

Alzheimer's Disease International
(federation of more than 100 member countries)
64 Great Suffolk St.
London, SEI OBK, United Kingdom
44-20-79810880   www.alz.co.uk

Lewy Body Disease

Lewy Body Disease Association
912 Killian Hill Rd., S.W.
Lilburn GA 30047
(404) 935-6444   www.lbda.org

Frontotemporal Degeneration

The Association for Frontotemporal Degeneration
Radnor Station Building 2, Ste. 320
290 King of Prussia Rd.
Radnor PA 19087
(866) 507-7222   www.theaftd.org

Frontotemporal Lobar Degeneration Association
PO Box 171221
San Antonio TX 78217
http://ftdabrainstorm.org

Creutzfeldt-Jakob Disease

Creutzfeldt-Jakob Disease Foundation
341 W. 38th St., Ste. 501
New York NY 10018
(800) 659-1991   www.cjdfoundation.org

Books by People with Alzheimer's Disease

Allen, Marjorie N., Susan Dublin, and Patricia J. Kimmerly. *A Look Inside Alzheimer's.* New York: Demos Health, 2012.

Bryden, Christine. *Who Will I Be When I Die?* London: Jessica Kingsley Publishers, 2012.

Bryden, Christine. *Dancing with Dementia: My Story of Living Positively with Dementia.* London: Jessica Kingsley Publishers, 2005.

Davis, Robert. *My Journey into Alzheimer's Disease.* Carol Stream, IL: Tyndale House Publishers, 1989.

DeBaggio, Thomas. *Losing My Mind: An Intimate Look at Life with Alzheimer's.* New York: The Free Press. 2002

Ferrari, Drew, Lorna Ferrari, and Leo C. Ferrari. *Different Minds: Living with Alzheimer, Disease.* New Brunswick, NJ: Goose Lane, 2005.

Henderson, Cary Smith, Jackie Henderson Main, Ruth D. Henderson, and Nancy Andrews. *Partial View: An Alzheimer's Journal.* Dallas, TX: Southern Methodist University Press, 1998.

McGowin, Diana Friel. *Living in the Labyrinth: A Personal Journey Through the Maze of Alzheimer's.* San Francisco, CA: Elder Books, 1993.

Mobley, Tracey. *Young Hope, The Broken Road.* Parker, CO: Outskirts Press, 2007.

Murray Alzheimer's Research and Education Program. *By Us For Us Guides.* A series of six guides created by a group of people with dementia. You can order the guides at: http://www.marep.uwaterloo.ca/products or call (519) 888-4567, ext. 36880.

Raushi, Thaddeus. *A View from Within.* Albany, NY: Northeastern New York Chapter, Alzheimer's Association, 2001.

Rose, Larry. *Show Me the Way to Go Home.* Forest Knolls, CA: Elder Books, 1995.

Rose, Larry. *Larry's Way: Another Look at Alzheimer's from the Inside.* Lincoln, NB: Universe, Inc., 2003.

Schneider, Charles. *Don't Bury Me…It Ain't Over Yet.* Bloomington, IN: Authorhouse Publishers, 2006.

Simpson, Robert, and Anne Simpson. *Through the Wilderness of Alzheimer's: A Guide in Two Voices.* Minneapolis, MN: Augsburg Fortress Publishers, 1999.

Summitt, Pat Head, and Sally Jenkins. *Sum It Up: A Thousand and Ninety-Eight Victories, a Couple of Irrelevant Losses, and a Life in Perspective.* New York: Crown Archetype, 2013.

Taylor, Richard. *Alzheimer's from the Inside Out.* Baltimore, MD: Health Professions Press, 2006. http://www.richardtaylorphd.com.)

Alzheimer's Disease and Dementia in Popular Films

Amour (2012). An award-winning foreign-language film set in France that follows the disturbing story of an older married couple facing the end of life. The woman suffers a series of strokes and her husband becomes consumed by her care.

A Separation (2011). Another award-winning foreign-language film set in Iran that portrays a young family torn by its devotion to an elder with Alzheimer's disease.

Win Win (2011). A struggling attorney (Paul Giamatti) takes on the guardianship of an elderly client with dementia in a desperate attempt to keep his practice afloat. When the client's teenage grandson runs away from home and shows up on his grandfather's doorstep, the attorney's life is turned upside down as his win–win proposition turns into something more complicated than he bargained for.

Barney's Version (2010). A hard-drinking hockey fanatic and television producer (Paul Giamatti) reflects on his successes and numerous failures as the final chapter of his own life comes sharply into focus.

Away from Her (2006). A woman with Alzheimer's disease (Julie Christie) voluntarily enters a care facility to avoid being a burden on her husband of fifty years. After a thirty-day separation, she has forgotten him and developed a relationship with another man.

The Savages (2007). Two estranged siblings (Laura Linney and Philip Seymour Hoffman) struggle to care their father with dementia and come to terms with each other in a tragic comedy.

Aurora Borealis (2005). A man with dementia (Donald Sutherland) requires more care than his wife (Louise Fletcher) can handle. They enlist the help of a home health aide and their grandson who forge a friendship as they care for him.

The Notebook (2004). Based on Nicholas Sparks' best-selling novel by the same name, a husband (James Garner) attempts to rekindle memories with his wife (Gena Rowlands) who lives in a nursing home.

Noel (2004). A daughter (Susan Sarandon) spends the Christmas holidays at a nursing home with her mother who has Alzheimer's disease and learns about redemption and forgiveness.

A Song for Martin (2001). Two musicians meet and marry in midlife, but soon after, they find out that he has Alzheimer's disease. This is a Swedish film with subtitles.

Iris: A Memoir of Iris Murdoch (2001). Based on the book *Elegy for Iris* by John Bayley, this is the true story of English novelist Iris Murdoch's Alzheimer's disease and the unconditional love of Bayley, her partner of forty years.

Index